A VOLUME IN THE SERIES

The Culture and Politics of Health Care Work

Edited by Suzanne Gordon *and* Sioban Nelson

A list of titles in this series is available at www.cornellpress.cornell.edu

COLLABORATIVE CARING

Stories and Reflections on Teamwork in Health Care

EDITED BY

SUZANNE GORDON,

DAVID L. FELDMAN, MD,

AND MICHAEL LEONARD, MD

ILR Press
an imprint of
Cornell University Press
ITHACA AND LONDON

First published 2014 by Cornell University Press

Printed in the United States of America

Library of Congress Cataloging-in-Publication Data

Collaborative caring : stories and reflections on teamwork in health care /
    edited by Suzanne Gordon, David L. Feldman, MD, Michael Leonard, MD.
        pages cm — (Culture and politics of health care work)
    Includes bibliographical references.
    ISBN 978-0-8014-5339-7 (cloth : alk. paper)
    1. Health care teams. I. Gordon, Suzanne, 1945– editor. II. Feldman, David L.,
editor. III. Leonard, Michael (Anesthesiologist), editor. IV. Jackson, Andrea
(Obstetrician). Learning to really listen. V. Series: Culture and politics of health
care work.
    R729.5.H4C66   2015
    362.106—dc23   2014024458

Cornell University Press strives to use environmentally
responsible suppliers and materials to the fullest extent
possible in the publishing of its books. Such materials include
vegetable-based, low-VOC inks and acid-free papers that
are recycled, totally chlorine-free, or partly composed of
nonwood fibers. For further information, visit our website
at www.cornellpress.cornell.edu.

Cloth printing   10 9 8 7 6 5 4 3 2 1

Contents

Collaborative Caring

Introduction

These days, teamwork is all the rage in health care. No matter where you look, there is talk of teams. There are interdisciplinary or interprofessional teams, medical teams and nursing teams, patient-centered teams and patients at the center of the team. We constantly hear that there is no "I" in the word "team," or else we find out how to put it back into the team through leadership. Listen to the buzz and you find that teamwork today isn't only for elite players—the quarterbacks and pitchers of health care—but is all-inclusive. Housekeepers, transporters, patient care assistants, and elevator operators—everyone is supposedly on the team, and it supposedly takes everyone to deliver patient care and enhance the patient experience.

In 1999, the Institute of Medicine launched the contemporary patient safety movement with *To Err Is Human*, which reported that each year almost 100,000 people die and 1.5 million are injured because of medical errors.[1] Its subsequent report in 2001, *Crossing the Quality Chasm*, argued that better teamwork and communication among all those who work in health care could vastly reduce that toll of injuries and deaths.[2] In 2013, the World Health Organization published its "Framework for Interprofessional Education and Collaborative Practice" and the *Lancet* its "Health Professionals for a New Century: Transforming Education to Strengthen Health Systems in an Interdependent World."[3]

Given the rhetoric about the importance of teamwork, one would think that health care institutions of every kind would have taken up the challenge to move from the traditional model of parallel play among intimate strangers (known in the trade as "siloed care") to a genuine teamwork model.[4] One would also think that this paradigm shift in the rhetoric would be reflected in both the facts on the ground and the statistics. When one looks at the statistics, however, there is

1

barely any positive movement in the number of patients harmed or killed in health care today. In fact, new studies document that the IOM's original estimate of 98,000 people killed each year from medical errors and injuries was a dramatic underestimation. Recent Medicare data tells us that more than 200,000 patients per year die as a result of avoidable medical harm, and we know one in three patients admitted to a US hospital suffers an adverse event there. Yet another report estimates the number of deaths to be between 220,000 and 440,000.[5] As for the facts on the ground, anecdotal reports reveal that—some pockets of excellent teamwork notwithstanding—teamwork in most health care settings is more of a dream than a reality. What explains this contrast between rhetoric and reality? We believe it's a failure to understand what teams are, how they are built, how they are led, how members on teams should really behave if genuine teamwork is to be realized, and how they are sustained over time.

There are many theoretical and conceptual books and countless articles that have explored issues of teamwork in general and teamwork in health care in particular. The editors, and many of the authors in this book, have read most, and have even written some of them. To tackle the issue of teamwork, we have, however, taken a different approach. Rather than write a theoretical book about what teamwork is, what it is not, where it exists in health care, what barriers prevent its implementation and how they can be removed, we have chosen instead to address these questions through narratives and reflections that vividly describe good teamwork as well as problems in creating, leading, and working on genuine teams. What we believe is too often lacking in the literature is a clear and compelling picture of what teamwork looks like on the ground, in the institutions where health care work is delivered and where teams play well, or don't play well, on a daily basis. The question we ask here is thus: What is the state of play in most health care institutions?

To describe the state of play, we have asked clinicians to write what we think of as "where the rubber hits the road" stories or reflections about the nature of teamwork in their own particular work setting. To gather these stories, we talked to many people in different health care disciplines. In the invitation for submissions we wrote the following: "We are seeking short, concise narratives that describe a concrete example in which you personally have been involved. The idea here is not to focus so much on the individual doctor-patient, nurse-patient, therapist-patient communication but the teamwork that was involved in ensuring that the standard of care was met or exceeded. If the patient or family was involved, so much the better. Stories can deal with interprofessional or intraprofessional teamwork. On balance, we would prefer to have more stories about interprofessional or occupational teamwork. Nonetheless, we recognize that interprofessional work depends on the ability to create teamwork within an occupation or profession. Stories involving support staff, such as housekeepers who spoke up about a patient safety issue, are definitely within the purview of this book. We would also welcome personal reflections that would enhance our understanding of either how to produce genuine teamwork or the obstacles that stand in its way."

When we extended our invitation, we deliberately asked people not to focus exclusively on the dyad of doctor-patient, nurse-patient, PT-patient relationship, which is what so much of the pedagogy on communication in health care has addressed. Although we have included stories by patients, and patients are involved in almost every story, we are convinced that no system of patient-centered care—or that claims it wants to put the patient at the center of the team—can succeed if all the rest of the players are flying solo and there is essentially no team on which the patient can, in fact, play. While good communication and teamwork among different groups, professions, and disciplines does not necessarily assure good communication and teamwork with patients, it is a necessary but insufficient condition for the genuine inclusion of the patient on the team, and, thus, the creation of patient-centered care.

Indeed, we would bet that poor communication and lack of teamwork (particularly what Suzanne Gordon terms "total communication meltdowns," or TCMs) are the foundation of patient harm. Even if such TCMs don't directly involve patients, if you look carefully, you will find that at the sharp end of such poor teamwork and communication is the patient who inevitably suffers from the existence of unresolved conflict, abuse, and other major and minor teamwork failures. Those who work in health care at every level often assert that their "professionalism" will somehow trump the fact that they have been told off, reamed out, ignored, or otherwise publically or privately disrespected and that they can function at an optimum level in spite of all manner of conflicts and problems. Health care managers and administrators are even more enamored of the myth that health care workers can just suck it up and perform with aplomb in spite of unmanageable workloads, fatigue, lack of support, simmering resentments, and outright conflicts as well as other assorted, unresolved problems.

This is a long-winded way of saying that although this book does not focus squarely on the patient and clinician-patient communication, its every word, comma, and semicolon is dedicated to the proposition that excellent intra- and interprofessional teamwork and communication among those who work in health care is the only avenue for putting the patient first and making health care safer and more cost effective.

People who work in many different areas in health care have written the stories in this book. Even the stories from the point of view of patients are written by patients who have a great deal of experience in health care, either as clinicians or researchers or both. Almost all the authors are identified by name. In one case, in which the author reported on a serious failure of teamwork, the author requested not to be identified, and we decided to include that anonymously written story. We can assure you that this is an expert practitioner who, for reasons that will be obvious when you read the story, worried about being disciplined if identifying details were printed.

We deliberately solicited these very "real world" stories because we wanted to move beyond theory to practice to show—rather than tell—readers what it takes to make a team, lead a team, and be a team member. We also wanted to show, rather than tell, how easy it is for smart people of very good will to defeat—or create—teamwork and thus quality patient care.

All of the essays in this book explore what the great Canadian sociologist Erving Goffman called the "backstage" and private spaces where culture manifests itself and where it is either reinforced or transformed. In Goffman's theories, front-stage spaces are those in which people present their idealized self or their ideals and the behaviors to which they aspire.[6] Spectators to front-stage exchanges, such as a speech about the necessity of teamwork, the presentation of a white paper on the need for civility and respect, or a workshop on conflict resolution, often extol, applaud, or assent—sometimes enthusiastically or sometimes grudgingly—to the ideas expressed. It is in backstage and private spaces—the discussions after the presentation that take place in the hallways, the behavior exhibited during the transfer of information (or lack of transfer of information) between putative team members, the way one deals with a suggestion or warning from a so-called subordinate—that we understand what issues need to be targeted or where change is actively occurring. Changing culture as it relates to teams from the front stage to these backstage and private spaces is the challenge in patient safety, interprofessional education, and practice.

Although this book is not a theoretical exploration of teamwork and its lack in health care, we do want to present a few basic definitions of what we consider to be teamwork, team intelligence, and several other key concepts without which teamwork is impossible. These concepts and definitions come to life in the stories we present.

When one asks about the state of play of teamwork—and how collaborative caring is—in health care the question that inevitably arises is "What in fact is a team?" When we looked up the etymology of the word "team" in the dictionary, we found that "team" first appeared in Old English and referred to a group of "draft animals that are yoked together to perform a task." The operative concept here is coordinated action. To be yoked together means that one can't move unless one's teammate cooperates and knows in what direction they're heading. "Team members" operating in silos are by definition not members of a team. Not only are they ineffective but also they work in a counterproductive manner.

One of the leading theorists and researchers in teamwork, the Harvard sociologist J. Richard Hackman, would call such groupings as teams "in name only." Hackman articulates five conditions of successful teamwork: "The team must be a real team, rather than a team in name only; it has a compelling direction for its work; it has an enabling structure that facilitates teamwork; it operates within a supportive organizational context; and it has expert teamwork coaching."[7]

Simply producing a good output (in this case quality patient care), Hackman cautions, is not enough to qualify as an example of successful teamwork. To be effective, a team or work group must satisfy three other requirements: It must produce an output that "meets the standards of quantity, quality, and timeliness of the people who receive, review, and/or use that output"; the process through which that output is produced must enhance "the capability of members to work together interdependently in the future"; and the process through which the team or group works must contribute "to the growth and personal well-being of team members."[8]

As David Feldman has written elsewhere, "Teams achieve competency when there is an optimal outcome and when team members feel good about the work they have done, can repeat the performance, and can teach their performance to others."[9] Scott Reeves and his colleagues have defined the concept of interprofessional teamwork to include the fact that those who work together on teams "don't only learn with and from each other but about the work that different members perform."[10] (We followed this guideline in choosing our stories and rejected several because the authors—say a physician— defined teamwork as handing a patient off to another professional— say a social worker—but could not describe, in their narratives, what, in fact, the social worker did with, or even for, the patient.)

Hackman's conceptualization of teams and teamwork has informed Gordon's notion of what she calls "team intelligence"—whose presence or absence is highlighted in every one of the stories in this book.[11]

Team intelligence is the active capacity of individual members of a team to learn, teach, communicate, reason, and think together, irrespective of their position in any hierarchy, in the service of realizing shared goals and a shared mission. Team intelligence has the following requisites:

- Team members must develop a shared team identity that allows them to articulate a shared mental model, shared language, and shared assumptions.
- Team members must be willing and able to share information, cross monitor, and coach all members of the team, as well as to solicit and take into account their input, no matter their position in the occupational hierarchy.

- Team members must understand one another's roles and work imperatives and how these mesh so that common goals can best be accomplished.
- Team members must help and support one another so that each individual member can perform his or her job efficiently and effectively.

One of our favorite definitions of teamwork comes from Edgar Schein's book *Helping*: "We do not typically think of an effective team as being a group of people who really know how to help each other in the performance of a task, yet that is precisely what good teamwork is—successful reciprocal help."[12] Schein also points out that two conditions must be met for people (and teams) to be receptive to input: first, the feedback must be respectful, so that no one loses face; and second, people must be given very specific advice that they can act on.

Another concept that is key to teamwork and the stories in this book has been well articulated by the cognitive anthropologist Edwin Hutchins—that is, the concept of "distributed cognition." As Hutchins explains:

> All divisions of labor, whether the labor is physical or cognitive in nature, require distributed cognition in order to coordinate the activities of the participants. Even a simple system of two men driving a spike with hammers requires some cognition on the part of each to coordinate his own activities with those of the other. When the labor that is distributed is cognitive labor, the system involves the distribution of two kinds of cognitive labor: the cognition that is the task and the cognition that governs the coordination of the elements of the task.[13]

In other words, you can't have a team and teamwork if you don't know and acknowledge that other people with whom you work—even if they perform what is perceived as lower-level work such as washing a floor or making a bed—know something, are doing something important, and have something to contribute and might actually discover information vital to patient care and safety. Members of a real team need to know not only what they are doing but also what their colleagues are doing, and they can't know this if they think the people they work with or who work around them are doing little of importance. (This means, of course, that they need to think about the people from the other professions and occupations with whom they work as colleagues working together with them to deliver patient care.) They also need to be mindful of what it takes to coordinate various tasks and activities.

Chris Argyris speaks to the importance of a work environment in which it is safe for workers to speak up, where workers have confidence they will receive feedback and their concerns will be acted on. In the absence of these conditions, he notes, even highly skilled people will arrive at work every day and abdicate responsibility for fixing problems.[14]

Last, but in this case most definitely not least, teamwork depends on psychological safety. This concept of psychological safety is interwoven into almost every story in this book. It was first described by Edgar H. Schein and Warren B. Bennis in *Personal and Organizational Change through Group Methods* where they argue that organizational and individual learning depends on something they call "unfreezing." To learn new behaviors or ideas and develop curiosity about human behavior and about themselves, people need to "unfreeze." To do this, they must feel psychologically safe within a particular group so that they can "take chances without fear and with sufficient protection." Learning new ideas and behaviors requires the ability to rock the boat, take risks, challenge a higher up, and stop playing it safe. None of this will happen if people are belittled, punished, humiliated, made fun of, ignored, abused, or otherwise disrespected. As Schein and Bennis write, psychologically safe organizations encourage provisional attempts and tolerate "failure without retaliation, renunciation, or guilt."[15]

Amy Edmondson emphasizes that psychological safety is essential to the creation of the kind of institutional learning that is a non-negotiable requirement of high-reliability organizations: "Psychological safety describes individuals' perceptions about the consequences of interpersonal risks in their work environment. It consists of taken-for-granted beliefs about how others will respond when one puts oneself on the line, such as by asking questions, seeking feedback, reporting a mistake, or proposing a new idea."[16]

A psychologically safe environment is thus one in which people feel they can ask a "dumb question," stop action when they identify a safety problem, or challenge a superior without fear of retaliation, humiliation, or disregard. This is the very heart of teamwork and team functioning. Good teamwork and safe care are not possible in the absence of psychological safety.

The stories in this book bring these concepts and many others to life as they are played out in the health care workplace. The word "play" has multiple meanings. One obviously is about enacting. The narratives in this book show how people act out their roles in a real-world context and how, in doing so, they can either transform or reproduce the status quo. Some of these stories describe particular incidents or activities; others are reflections, which are also key to teamwork and a kind of mental replaying that allows us to learn from our mistakes.

"Play" also suggests activity that is repeated over and over again—a sports team *plays* a game, musicians *play* a piece of music, actors *play* a role and rehearse their lines. In order to play well together, however, those who perform the activity together have to be serious enough to devote time to group practice, rehearsal, warm-up, and follow-through. (How often do health care teams do any of this?)

To consider the state of play and whether or not caring is, in fact, collaborative, as this book does, it is also necessary to encompass the varieties of play—parallel, cooperative, competitive—that are common in health care settings today. It must take into account the knowledge that teamwork is dynamic and evolving. In settings where health care is moving toward a new paradigm of collaboration, as we see in most of these stories, we find that patients are safer and those who work in health care more satisfied. In stories in which people work together on true teams, patients are viewed not as abstractions (as in we love the ideal of the patient, just not the patient in front of us) or as objects of medical action but as actual participants in the drama and activity. Where only parallel play rather than actual collaborative teamwork is the norm, resentment and conflicts fester, while patients are overshadowed and seem, in some instances, to be more an afterthought.

To capture the nature of genuine collaborative caring on real teams we have divided the book into eight parts, each of which has a brief introduction that highlights its main take-home messages. Part 1 consists of stories that illustrate excellent teamwork. Each one is almost a textbook illustration of Hackman's definition of teamwork and of the cultivation of team intelligence and is grounded in an understanding of distributed cognition as well as the need for psychological safety. Part 2, on poor or nonexistent teamwork, is its antithesis and shows us what happens when the non-negotiables of teamwork and team intelligence are missing. The picture is not a pretty one. Part 3 describes the patient's experience of the nonfunctioning "team." These stories all too often reflect an environment—even in institutions that tout their "patient-centered care"—in which patients are invisible as human beings. This produces a void at the center of patient-centered care. When care is patient centered, as Julia Hallisy, Michael Leonard, and Catherine Skowronsky show in their contributions, it is only because clinicians are deeply reflective and work hard to create the kind of environment in which patients can be included in decisions.

Part 4 builds on our argument about teamwork to document what happens when institutions and individuals create environments that are psychologically safe. Discovering how to create such environments—and what specifically to do or say in dynamic situations often punctuated by crises—is central to unlocking the mysteries of teamwork and building sustainable teams that fulfill the three tenets of teamwork outlined by Hackman. Part 5, similarly, demonstrates that coaching and learning are critical to the dynamics of teamwork and to the constant refinement of team practice. Hospitals and other health care institutions can put staff through TeamSTEPPS and other training programs, but if there are no coaches who can cross monitor and help others develop and refine their team intelligence, little genuine teamwork will result from even the best intentions and efforts.

Part 6 looks at a new approach to patient advocacy. Each profession in health care claims to be doing what is best for the patient. All too often, this excludes working with those in other professions or occupations—or with the patient—to actually plan and coordinate care. In this part, we show what happens when patient advocacy is a collective activity. This understanding of the relationship between collective activity and quality patient care leads us to our penultimate section. Part 7 examines the barriers to teamwork. It is by now commonly accepted that health care professionals and workers function in silos. We would go even further and argue that the professions have been socialized to define themselves as working in opposition to one another. Their very professional self-definitions and identity, their modes of payment, their promotional and other reward structures are part of a larger organizational and cultural universe that discourages interprofessional—and sometimes even intraprofessional—collaboration and cooperation. Toxic hierarchies discourage a physician from attending to concerns from other professionals, such as a nurse, and people who work on the lowest rungs of the socially constructed health care ladder are almost entirely off the radar. The rigid hierarchies that emerge from this kind of professional and occupational infrastructure poison efforts to reconfigure care and must be directly addressed and deconstructed if people across all professions and occupations are to work effectively on teams.

Part 8 ends on the good news that some institutions are struggling valiantly to do precisely that. Stories that describe these beginning or successful and ongoing efforts at culture change illustrate what it really means to engage in the sustained work of transforming how people behave in a department, a large institution, or even an entire system. In these stories we see that the commitment to change must not only be supported at the top but also at the bottom; staff at all levels must lead and support change. The complex interaction between top-level institutional team leaders and frontline team members is well articulated in these stories. Indeed, they illustrate the point that Robert Ginnett has made when discussing the components of the aviation safety model of "crew resource management," which is that "you are not a leader if you have no followers."[17]

We believe the stories and reflections in this book will enhance our growing understanding of the problems that must be addressed and solved in health care. Many of the stories we include have been chosen—quite deliberately—because they highlight what happens in backstage and private spaces after enthusiasm for the principles and theories of teamwork and interprofessionalism have been expressed. These stories help us understand how, in those out-of-the-way spaces, teamwork is either enhanced or defeated and help us see the behaviors that need to be enacted if teamwork and patient safety are to become a reality. Although we suggest some of the take-home lessons from these stories, this book is not a manifesto: we hope to show rather than tell. As you read about other people's experiences, we hope you will gain insight into the work of those in health care with whom you are less familiar. We also hope some of these stories will help to illuminate the complexities that need to be addressed on the way forward.

Part 1

PLAYING ON A REAL TEAM

It seems almost too obvious to state, but effective team-work and communication in a collaborative environment is the very foundation of the delivery of safe, high-quality patient care.[1] Because so many studies on patient safety make this clear, one would think that genuine teamwork, excellent communication, and collaboration would be the norm in health care; that everyone who works in health care, in any capacity, would already be trained to work on a genuine team either as leader or assertive member; and that showcasing good teamwork in a book like this would be unnecessary.

Unfortunately, there are also many studies that document that teamwork, respect, and civility are more of an aspiration than a reality in the current health care environment. As Francis A. Rosinia recounts in part 8, when Tulane Medical Center asked its staff whether they believed in teamwork and respect, the majority of those surveyed said of course they did. When asked if they felt they were respected in the workplace and worked on real teams, the majority responded in the negative. Tulane is not unique. Those who work in health care have been socialized into an individual-expert model grounded in the expectation that smart, skilled people perform flawlessly and manage risk effectively. According to this way of thinking, people will act rationally in the most stressful circumstances and, if experts, they will rarely make mistakes.

Decades of research in human factors now documents that these assumptions are largely invalid. As the title of the Institute of Medicine's report on medical errors and injuries sums it up, to err is human.[2] Effective teamwork is essential, given the complexity of clinical care and chance for error. Currently, one in three hospital patients has something happen to them that you and I wouldn't want to happen to us, and 6 percent of patients are seriously enough harmed in the hospital that they need to stay longer and go home with a temporary or permanent disability.[3] Skill in the clinical setting does not lead to infallibility, nor does it translate into the kind of team intelligence that allows people to be both effective team leaders and members.

Fortunately, new models of leadership are emerging. These models do not involve expert individuals exerting either command or total control of the work process. As we see in the stories in part 1, high-quality leadership involves utilizing all the information available and making decisions based on the needs and concerns of everyone on the team—including the patient. Although there has been an increasing focus on "emotional intelligence" as a function of effective leadership, this concept is too often interpreted as simply learning to listen. Genuine team leaders, however, do more than listen; they solicit input from those whom they are leading, and they respond to that input, not simply hear it. They establish shared mental models and a shared language, and they clarify roles and assumptions. Perhaps most important, they do not regard the input of "subordinates" as challenges to their status or authority but rather as the expression of legitimate concerns about patient safety and work organization. The kind of mature leaders such as Philip Levitt, whom we see in action here, understand that they are fallible and thus need to work with assertive team members who can be counted on—indeed expected—to do the kind of critical cross monitoring described in his story.[4]

The expectation of cross monitoring is just one of the agreed on behaviors that characterize an effective team; such a team also establishes clear measures that allow team members to know how they are performing. In the TeamSTEPPS program, for example, an entire section is devoted to "mutual support," which is described as "backup behavior" that is "critical to the social and task performance of teams and essentially involves helping other team members perform their tasks."[5] Structured communication models including huddles, briefings, SBAR,[6] and similar techniques provide consistency and predictability in communication among team members. Good teams also acknowledge that conflict—like making mistakes—is inevitable. Whether they are leaders or members, those who work in real teams have been taught how to deal constructively with such conflict. This does not mean avoiding conflict but rather utilizing it to create learning on an individual and institutional level.[7]

Of course, good teamwork is all about relationships and trust. In the best-case scenario, real teams have been built with intentionality that is reinforced by systematic training and developed over years. In a dynamic health care environment, however, people can't always work in relationships that have been cultivated over months, much less decades. To create both a safe work environment and safe care, mindful team members must practice with people with whom they may have never worked.[8] This is why teamwork skills must be taught at all levels and revisited regularly.

In aviation, as Captain Chesley "Sully" Sullenberger explains, regular teamwork training and practice over an entire career makes it possible for people who have never worked together to quickly form teams capable of astonishing feats:

> Almost paradoxically, it was our training and culture of making the routine predictably reliable, building and leading a team (taking a team of experts and creating an expert team), having well-understood roles and responsibilities to our passengers and to each other, being schooled in the consistent application of best practices, using clear communication with a well-defined vocabulary where a single word (brace) could be rich with meaning and trigger team actions, and managing workload and error that enabled us to successfully handle a sudden challenge of a lifetime. Because aviation has built such a robust and resilient safety system in which we operate, it was a firm foundation on which we could, in 208 seconds, take what we did know, apply it in a new way, and solve a problem we'd never seen before. That, to me, is treating successfully a very "sick" situation full of complexity.[9]

The fact that a group of people, unfamiliar with one another five days earlier, managed to become hyperorganized in a matter of minutes, make a decision to land on the Hudson River, and get everyone off the plane and to safety without serious injury, is testament to the value of mindful *practice*. And here we use the word "practice" in the full sense of the term—putting an activity or skill into practice because a group has practiced together that set of activities and skills over and over again. Sometimes people practice with the same group of people; sometimes with different people. Nonetheless, the fact that they have practiced teamwork skills and mastered teamwork concepts means they can form teams quickly, like Sullenberger and his crew did in January 2009. This was a perfect illustration of the phenomenon Hackman describes—that collaborative teamwork not only produces discrete episodes in which people work well together and achieve good outcomes but also each of these discrete episodes is a building block in the larger edifice of ongoing team relationships and intelligence. The next episode of teamwork may include the same cast of characters or it may involve people who have never met before.

Good teamwork thus involves:

- treating everyone with respect;
- creating the kind of psychological safety that allows anyone, at any level, to freely speak up and voice concerns;
- knowing the plan of care for the patient and adjusting it appropriately;
- including the patient and the patient's family as valuable members of the team;
- learning together from mistakes;
- recognizing the value of voice-to-voice and face-to-face communication;
- refusing to confuse cross-monitoring with insubordination; and
- actively soliciting the concerns of others.

Teams that get all this right consistently deliver great care and fulfill the trust that sick patients and their families place in those who work in the health care system.

Learning to Really Listen

Andrea Jackson

When I was chief resident in obstetrics and gynecology at a teaching hospital in the Northeast, I learned a lesson that has totally transformed my practice. I was covering labor and delivery (L & D) at night. A patient, who was about six months into her pregnancy, was admitted after having a cervical cerclage placed. Her cervix was short and a little bit open, so we put a stitch through her cervix to keep it closed so she would not deliver prematurely. After this procedure we kept her in the hospital for observation to make sure that she recovered well from the procedure and didn't develop an infection.

Several hours after her admission, her nurse, who had had at least ten years of L & D experience, approached me. She said that she was concerned that the patient was in the very early phases of developing an infection and told me that I needed to remove her cerclage. I was immediately skeptical. The patient had just had her procedure; the physician who placed the cerclage did this routinely; and I didn't really think she had an infection. But to please the nurse—and really just to get her off my back—I went and evaluated the patient. The patient complained of some discomfort in her uterus and belly, but when I looked at her vital signs they were all normal: no fever, no elevated heart rate, no elevated fetal heart rate. I thought the discomfort was normal postoperative pain—what we would call uterine irritability. I wasn't concerned.

When I told the nurse what I thought, she became visibly upset. She again told me that the patient was going to develop an infection and insisted that I needed to remove her cerclage. At that point, I was trying to come up with a compromise and said I would come back and check on her in an hour. If she was worse, we could then readdress removing the cerclage.

At that point the nurse said, "You're a chief. You need to learn how to make a decision. You need to either shit or get off the pot."

Once she said that, I walked away because I didn't want to keep escalating what was clearly becoming a very contentious conversation. I was nonetheless upset because I felt she wasn't trusting my clinical knowledge. And, although I hate to admit it now, my response was also influenced by the feeling that she was not being sufficiently respectful of the fact that I was the physician and had a lot of medical knowledge.

During this standoff, someone spoke to the charge nurse, who appeared on the scene and suggested that the attending be called in. Fine, I thought, okay, whatever.

The attending quickly arrived. She asked both me and the nurse to explain the clinical situation and then went in to examine the patient herself. When she came out, she said she agreed with me. The patient's symptoms seemed very vague and "subjective." There were no hard numbers to quantify her condition and thus unambiguously validate the nurse's concern. However, the attending agreed with the nurse: something was going on. She specifically asked the nurse why she was so concerned about this patient. The attending physician's tone was not defensive, and she spoke to her as a colleague and with genuine curiosity.

The nurse quickly explained that over the past month the L & D service had had a rash of patients like this one. They were preterm; they expressed vague subjective complaints; and all of them had developed serious infections that required—at least in some cases—admission to the ICU.

The attending did a great job. She validated my clinical judgment and what I saw, which was that the patient's symptoms were indeed vague and ambiguous. But she agreed with the nurse. There was a possibility that this patient was developing an infection and that the risks of that outweighed the benefits of keeping the cerclage in. The attending told me to remove the cerclage, which I did.

The patient was kept in the hospital. While she didn't develop an infection and deliver immediately, over the next day, she developed a fever and tachycardia (her heart rate went up)—objective signs of an infection. The nurse had been right.

What I realized in reflecting on this was that the nurse and I both needed some lessons in communication. For someone with her level of experience, she could certainly have realized that, as an experienced

L & D nurse in a teaching hospital, she could have perhaps stepped into my shoes and understood that I was trying to find my way as a physician learning on the job. At the same time, I came to realize that I didn't help matters much, because in the kind of hierarchical antiteam system I'd been trained in, I quickly became as concerned about my stature and authority as about what we should do for the patient. When the attending came down and spoke to both of us, she managed to uncover both of our points of view, which neither of us had conveyed well to each other. She asked the nurse the question, I should have asked, which was, "Why are you so concerned about this patient?"

Although it took a while, the nurse and I eventually talked about this incident. We both apologized for our actions. In doing so, the nurse reiterated what the attending had uncovered, which was that she had taken care of many patients who had later gotten sick and recognized the writing on the wall. I apologized to her for getting so defensive and not listening to her. I acknowledged that I had started off the whole encounter by not really giving any weight to her concern. I saw the patient just to get the nurse off my back. We ended up working well together over the next year.

That interaction informed more than my relationship with one particular RN. It affected how I interact with nurses in a variety of situations and practice settings. Recently, I was working in a family planning clinic. I had finished a procedure, and one of the nurses was doing an ultrasound on the patient. I thought the procedure had gone well, so I was packing up my instruments and was about to leave the room when I looked back and saw that the nurse was still scanning the patient's abdomen. I knew what she was concerned about: she was worried that the procedure wasn't complete. But I was confident that it was.

For about one moment, I almost left the room and didn't address what I knew was going on. Then I remembered lessons learned and turned around and said, "Kim, are you concerned about something?"

At first she said, "No."

I saw the look on her face and how closely she was concentrating on the ultrasound, so I went back and sat down and said, "Kim, point to the area on the ultrasound that you're worried about." I was very careful to use a tone that was curious, pleasant, and respectful. "It's okay," I assured her, "I really want you to tell me if you are concerned about something."

She showed me what she was concerned about on the ultrasound. She was a new nurse in the clinic and so was clearly a bit worried about her judgment. When she showed me the area of concern, it turned out that it was normal anatomy. I explained to her that this was a normal part of the uterus, but I could tell she was a little hesitant or unclear, so I took a curette and placed it inside the uterus and both of us were able to see on the ultrasound that what she was concerned about was actually on the outside of the uterus. With that, I could tell she was visibly relieved, so I left the room, and the patient was fine.

At the end of the day Kim approached me and told me how much she appreciated my taking her concerns seriously. I again told her that even though, in this instance, I was "right," I valued her expertise and wanted her to feel comfortable in the future voicing any concerns about patient care to me. "I know there will be a time when I'm not right because it's happened before and will again," I told her.

Looking at the ultrasound with Kim took only, at the most, two more minutes. But taking those two minutes was critical. Our goal is to provide excellent patient care. We now know that the only way we can provide excellent patient care is through teamwork, which means recognizing and respecting the expertise each of us brings. Today there's a lot of lip service to this, but sometimes, in our rush to get things done, we don't actually do what it takes to make teamwork happen.

Kim and I love working together and always try to get paired up. Taking time to work on teamwork provides many rewards. One, of course, is more satisfying workplace relationships. I am convinced that this working on team dynamics also improves the level of care we provide our patients. We have to have this level of rapport with one another to give high-quality care.

· · ·

Andrea Jackson, MD is an obstetrician/gynecologist at San Francisco General Hospital and is Assistant Professor of Obstetrics, Gynecology, and Reproductive Medicine at University of California, San Francisco (UCSF) School of Medicine.

Sea Change

Philip Levitt

When I was a neurosurgery resident in the early 1970s, I read *Corporation Man* by Sir Antony Jay. In it Jay tells the story of a period when he was responsible for a live nightly TV news program on the BBC. The entire show was run by a small, insular group that he headed. There were directors, writers, researchers, and news anchors. It was a hectic, high-pressure undertaking. Jay called it the best professional experience of his life. It was special to him because everyone made contributions *outside* his or her area of expertise. Everyone listened to everyone else. The experts in their fields knew more about and could be creative in their specialties; nonetheless, everyone was allowed to contribute ideas. This was in part because the experts sometimes missed things. The results of listening to others were consistently beneficial to the objective of the group.

Jay compared his team to an imagined primitive human hunting band. Each member had his or her own strengths and skills, and survival was based on the sharing of ideas, shared responsibility, and teamwork. Jay deplored treating one's subordinates as interchangeable ciphers whose opinions and suggestions were never sought. He knew that in any particular aspect of a project there was likely a group member with greater skill or judgment or a more inspired plan.

The environment I worked in was nothing like Jay's. I was trained and then practiced in the self-reliant captain-of-the-ship model of neurosurgery. My professor was an autocratic old-school academic leader who got outstanding surgical results. Although he preached cooperation and communication, he was a less-than-perfect role model. He would bawl out a nurse on rounds in front of the residents, patient, and family and would be intolerant of the residents' raising questions about patient care.

In the community hospitals where I worked after my residency, the patient care paradigm was one private practitioner and one nurse to each patient. Occasional consultants chipped in with their narrowly crafted advice, staying entirely within their own area of expertise and rarely communicating other than leaving notes in the patient's chart.

In spring 1998, I returned to caring for patients with severe head injuries after a seven-year hiatus. Two trauma centers in our county had started up during that period. The emergency rooms at my usual hospitals were legally obliged to send all badly head-injured patients to the centers, and I never had to see them. One of the centers was at St. Joe's where, over the seven years, I had gradually moved my practice. I figured that the four or five twenty-four-hour on-call periods each month would be no big deal, so I signed on. Even though I'd had a seven-year break from treating head injuries, I reckoned, I'm a Bellevue-trained neurosurgeon, and I saw a lot of trauma at my other hospitals until they opened the trauma centers. Getting in and out of a head is the same whether it's a tumor, an aneurysm, or a traumatic blood clot, so I haven't had any atrophy of the required skills.

I never could have predicted, however, the ego-deflating episode that occurred one Saturday night, two months after my enlisting. Maybe it's good to be shaken out of one's complacency once in a while, but it still hurts when I think how close my patient and I came to disaster.

The patient was fourteen. She had told her mother she was sleeping over at a girlfriend's house, but at 9 p.m. she was sitting in the rear of a car driven by a nineteen-year-old boy she had just met and his buddy who sat in the front passenger seat. Her girlfriend sat beside her. There were no seatbelts in the rear, and the doors weren't locked. When the crash occurred she was asleep. She was thrown from the car onto the pavement. She came into the trauma ER unconscious with a blood pressure of zero. A CT of her brain showed a tiny amount of bruising. Her abdomen was full of blood on CT, and the spleen looked ruptured. The on-call trauma doctor, Rick Sanchez, took her right to surgery to open her belly. He had the nurses call me to put an intracranial pressure monitor through the right front part of her skull as she lay intubated on the operating table. The pressure was 5, which is normal. Abnormal pressures are 20 or above.

"You want me to retract for you?" I asked the trauma doctor. I was fifteen years his senior and had not assisted in the OR for ten years. "I once had a surgical internship. I think I can still do it."

"Sure. If you don't mind, scrub in."

I assisted while he took quarts of blood out of her belly and removed her ruptured spleen. Her blood pressure started to come up as I was leaving. Sanchez thanked me as I exited.

I went home. It was about 1 a.m. when Sanchez called me about her.

"Her intracranial pressure is 25 now on the monitor."

"That's high, but her CT was nearly normal. All she had was a small contusion."

"Wouldn't you want to get another CT anyway to explain why the pressure became elevated, just to be safe?"

"Sure," I said sheepishly. What he said made perfect neurosurgical sense.

She had a big epidural hematoma, a massive, expanding, deadly clot compressing her brain. The difference from the earlier CT scan was like day and night. An epidural comes from a torn artery that lies partly within the bone of the skull. A "mere" skull fracture in a bad place does the tearing.

We both had figured out how this had happened. The artery tore when she hit the pavement but didn't bleed because she had no blood pressure. That is why the initial CT was nearly normal, giving me, at least, a false sense of assurance that her head was not a problem. However, when the trauma doctor restored the blood pressure by taking out her spleen, the open artery in her head began to bleed briskly, and a big clot grew between her skull and her brain. Neither of us had ever seen anything like this before, neither somebody surviving after a BP of zero with a ruptured spleen, nor a delayed appearance on a CT of a big epidural clot. Sanchez assisted me with the craniotomy to remove the clot. She throve.

Two years later it was confession time. I was speaking with a crackerjack trauma nurse, one of the people who held the whole service together.

I said, "You know Rick saved my career that night. If the medical examiner had found a big epidural clot in that girl I would have been toast. I'll always be grateful."

"We would never have let anything like that happen to you, Dr. Levitt."

Three years later, when I was appointed chief of neurosurgery, I had the opportunity to verbalize in committees what I had learned from being part of the trauma service. My insight had begun with the night that Rick Sanchez thought of getting the extra CT on the kid with the ruptured spleen. I suspect that everyone got tired of hearing me say my bit. Here is what I would say with a lot of variation, month after month to the nurses, techs, and doctors at the trauma service meeting.

"We have at least two teams of doctors and nurses making rounds on these patients every day. The two most active teams, the trauma doctors and their nurses and the neurosurgeon and the neurosurgery nurse, are present for rounds at the same time every morning in the same ICU. There's an ICU nurse assigned to each patient. That's another set of eyes. The other consultants come in and out and they talk to us. We each check each other's work. I have to look at the vital signs and lab results. The nurses and the trauma docs get the reports and images on the head injury patients, and they let me know if there's something unexpected in the head and what's going on in the rest of the patient's body. I know the pO_2 and pCO_2 of the patients, and sometimes I'm the first to tell them that something is out of whack with their respiratory function. I tell them what's going on with the brain, and we discuss whether our treatment approaches are compatible. Everybody questions everything. A neurosurgical nurse whom we all know follows me around like Jiminy Cricket. If I can't justify what I'm doing to her, I have to rethink it. The key to running a safe service is redundancy, the more the merrier. But we're not really redundant. All of us are necessary to the survival of such very sick patients. We pick up on each other's mistakes and omissions, and that's why we have good outcomes.

"Also, look around you. There are twenty people sitting at this table; all the chairs against the wall are filled, and there are people standing. We don't get attendance like this for any other committee meeting of the hospital. I think that says a lot about the morale on the trauma service."

Another change occurred in my professional life, in its own way more surprising than the rest. As a result of signing up for the trauma center, I was working with a group of three neurosurgeons who formerly had been my competitors, doctors who saw my mistakes while rendering second opinions while I saw theirs. We reviewed one another's charts for the sieve-like peer review committees that were sworn to silence but broadcast our mistakes as juicy bits of physician-to-physician gossip. We heard comments made about one another by patients and other doctors—the good and the bad. There wasn't much collegiality in our prior state, and there was a lot of resentment and envy, things that are inevitable given human nature and the century-old private practice system we inherited. That mostly changed when we worked together for six years. We meshed beautifully and trusted and liked one another. Most of us retained our private practices, but it was not like before. We were colleagues for the first time. We rotated every twenty-four hours, and two of us signed out to each other at 7 a.m. every morning and got to talk to each other a lot about patient care and our philosophies of approaching difficult problems. Important bits and pieces of our personal lives stole into our conversations.

They had high professional standards. And the nurses and trauma doctors we interacted with were true colleagues. I look back at those six years as the best for me professionally by far. Six years out of thirty-two. I suspect most docs don't get that much, based on the grim burnout statistics. You have to be lucky. The doctors I enjoyed working with so much had a deep wellspring of good will and democratic idealism. I don't believe they were taught that in medical school.

· · ·

PHILIP LEVITT, MD is a retired Neurosurgeon and former Chief of Staff and Chief of Neurosurgery of two hospitals in Palm Beach County, Florida—St. Mary's and JFK Memorial. He writes on patient safety for internet publications and medical journals; his latest article is "Staying Out of Trouble" in the *Journal of Digital Imaging*. He was the recipient of the Hans Berger prize of the American EEG Society for laboratory investigations of the effects of subarachnoid hemorrhage on cortical activity.

A Genuine Collaboration

Jay A. Perman and Elsie M. Stines

More and more physicians today are employing nurse practitioners (NPs) in their practices. In many of these settings, the typical practice model too often involves the NP doing what the physician chooses not to do. The NP sees more routine cases—say, uncomplicated new patients, well-child visits, sore throats, or upper respiratory infections—and in this the NP is supervised by the MD. Or the NP may do the follow-up visits for more complicated patients after the physician has determined their diagnosis and course of treatment. The general rule is that the more complicated the patient, the less involved the NP. It is the physician who decides what kind of patient the NP will see.

Although many would consider this to be an interprofessional practice, because two different professions are working, if not together, at least in proximity, this model maintains the traditional physician hierarchy. The physician often conceptualizes the NP as working for him or her—and sometimes even refers to the NP as "my" nurse practitioner.

We think of the model we have elaborated over our decade of practice in the field of pediatric gastroenterology in a very different way. For us it is a partnership rather than a hierarchical relationship. Rather than Dr. Perman referring to NP Stines or thinking of NP Stines as "his" NP and as working for him, we work with each other. We are colleagues and refer to each other as such, as in "my colleague Dr. Perman" and "my colleague Nurse Stines" or "Ms. Stines." This is in spite of the fact that Dr. Perman taught NP Stines a great deal about pediatric gastroenterology from the medical point of view. At this point in our relationship, neither partner is teacher or learner. We teach and learn from each other.

This is not an abstract exercise in political correctness. It's about better patient care and even makes economic sense in that we can see more patients. Fundamentally, this model reflects our recognition that the more complicated a case gets the more we benefit from working not separately but together. This commitment to colleagueship or partnership, in turn, is embedded in how we deal with our patients in a practice that, over the years, has attracted referrals that some might call "diagnostic dilemmas" from around the state of Maryland and beyond. Others might be less flattering, sadly referring to the children and families we see as "crocks." That is, our young patients are sometimes sent to us because someone believes they are school phobic. Sometimes other physicians have been concerned that a mother is embellishing her child's symptoms. Whatever the reason for the referral, patients come because initial attempts at diagnosis and therapy failed; the belly (most commonly) still hurts. And the referral occurred because either the pediatrician wasn't sure about the patient or family or the parents weren't sure about the pediatrician. Or perhaps everyone had their doubts, and the physician just didn't have the time to manage the issue further. So off they come to Stines and Perman.

And here's what happens when they arrive. One of us will usually see the patient and family on their first visit. It could be either one. Then we talk together about the patient, and then we see the patient together when we have decided on a diagnosis and treatment plan. Seeing patients together, after one of us has seen a patient alone, is very useful. As one of us is talking, a family member is listening and discovers that we have misunderstood something or that they have not told us everything and have left out an important detail. Or one of us notices something that the other didn't.

When people call us with an exceedingly complicated diagnostic dilemma, we will see a patient together on that first-time visit. We recognize that the more complicated the case, the better it is to have four eyes, four ears, and two brains from the start. Dr. Perman might say to NP Stines, "Let's hear this together," or visa versa. If one of us sees a very complex patient and then repeats the long and complicated history to the other, the risk is that nuance and detail will be lost. Moreover, as mentioned, while one of us is talking to the patient or family, the other can be observing how they react. This can provide enormous amounts of information. Sometimes very complex cases require not only the two of us but other people as well, pharmacists, social workers, dieticians or nutritionists, and/or psychologists—not working serially in isolation but working together with the patient and family.

Working together doesn't only mean seeing a patient and family together at times. It always involves a negotiation. In our practice, Dr. Perman does not dictate the diagnosis and treatment because he is the physician, nor does NP Stines simply step back because she's the NP. We discuss what is the best diagnostic approach. If NP Stines disagrees with the recommendation and says we should not do it, Dr. Perman does not get an automatic override. We talk it through. In doing so, we have never reached a stalemate. Dr. Perman might say, "Elsie this doesn't make sense," and she may say, "But, Jay, it doesn't make sense to do it that way either." We are not the only ones who negotiate; we always include the family. In fact, there are times when the family may intervene and say, "You know what, we don't like a more aggressive approach. We prefer a step-wise approach. If we're first going to try a therapy, we need more investigation."

We also do not hesitate to disagree politely with the patient and family present. Dr. Perman may detect that NP Stines doesn't agree with him and will sometimes say, "I can see that Nurse Stines has some concerns here." Or one of us will say, "Let's think this out to- gether" or "I need my colleague or colleagues to help me make a decision." And then we will openly discuss our concerns in front of the patient and family. Some people might object that if we do not show a united front and show that we disagree that this will scare either the patient or family. We have never found this to be the case. In fact, if patients and families see that we can politely and construc- tively disagree, then that gives them permission to raise their con- cerns as well.

Let us give you an illustrative example of how we take care of our patients. Ten-year-old David from the Eastern Shore of Maryland was referred for abdominal pain. He missed a great deal of school and eventually was not attending school at all. We were sure there was a disease process; certainly we needed more diagnostic and lab- oratory testing and probably medication as well. NP Stines went into the room and introduced herself to both David and David's mother and explained that she was a pediatric nurse practitioner and that she worked with Dr. Perman and together they would be caring for David. After she obtained a very complex and detailed history, she performed a head-to-toe physical exam. Stines told the mother and David what she thought was concerning about the history and physical exam, but said she was going to speak with Dr. Perman and other colleagues. Together, with the family, the *team* would decide the plan.

NP Stines then headed back to the conference room, which is a common area where providers and other members of our team—a dietician, medical students, the behavioral psychologist Ramasamy Manikam, and a nurse—gather to discuss patients. After providing the history and physical exam to Dr. Perman and the team, we discussed possible diagnoses and what the next steps would be. Dr. Perman and NP Stines together headed back to the exam room to speak with David and his mother. Dr. Perman went over the key points in the history and physical exam, and together we discussed our concerns and recommended the next steps.

During our discussions with the family, Dr. Perman would ask if NP Stines agreed and if she thought we should do anything different. We asked David and his mother if they had any questions or concerns and if there were any obstacles that would prevent them from agreeing to the plan. At the end of the visit, Dr. Perman said to the family, "Nurse Stines and I have been working together for a while, and we have very similar practice styles, and we always communicate any concerns to each other."

A follow-up visit was scheduled to discuss results and to see if medications that were prescribed were helping. Although all of David's test results were negative, he continued not to attend school. Because behavioral and physical issues are often intermingled, our message to David was: "We've never seen any child where it was 100 percent organic or 100 percent functional. It's really some part of each, and our approach is to work with you on both, sometimes more in the behavioral and coping spheres, and especially if the picture changes, sometime more with therapeutic agents. And David, you are going to school, and you will do the best you can."

We asked David's mother if she could update us in two weeks and let us know how things were going with David and how he had been adjusting going back to school. We told David and his mother that we wanted to see them back in three to four weeks.

David became more functional; he went to school for a few hours each day and eventually was able to attend the whole day. When David would come in for his follow-up visits, we would assess his progress and decide together the goals for David and the information we would convey. One of us would begin the visit, and the other would drop in to say hello and reinforce the plan.

One day, with an admiring smile on her face, David's mother told us, "You two work so well together!" It was meant as a compliment to our practice style, of course, but it meant something more to us. We realized that this impression she had of our practice was one of the many elements that helped her child. She believed she could trust this team, albeit small, of professionals specially attuned to rehabilitate her son and provide relief for her.

In our years of working together we have had many patients like this. We have approached them in much the same manner, but sometimes very fortunately aided by Ramasamy Manikam. He is sheer Mr. Practical—that's the way he advises and also may reinforce what we work out together as the plan of care.

We have had several opportunities to leverage ourselves as a nurse practitioner–physician team with families who seem to understand what we bring individually and together as partners and colleagues to their care. We feel that the quality of care we deliver is higher as a result of this partnership. It certainly makes it more satisfying for us to deliver care through this model. In fact, we cannot imagine working in any other way.

. . .

JAY A. PERMAN, MD is President of the University of Maryland, Baltimore. He is a pediatric gastroenterologist with longstanding interests in team-based professional practice. He conducts a weekly clinic in which patients and families are evaluated and treated by an interprofessional faculty together with students in nursing, medicine, pharmacy, dentistry, social work, and law.

ELSIE M. STINES, CRNP, RN is a Pediatric Nurse Practitioner specializing in Pediatric Gastroenterology and Nutrition. She directs the President's

Clinic at the University of Maryland, Baltimore, which is an interprofessional health education and practice program providing intensive experiences in team-based care for health science, law, and social work students. She also serves as project director for special initiatives undertaken by the president of the University of Maryland, Baltimore.

Out of Sight, Out of Mind

Martyn Diaper

I have been a general practitioner for over seventeen years. Working in a small market city not quite an hour from London has introduced me to patients from all walks of life, and I have enjoyed becoming part of that community.

Seven or eight years ago, a new patient, Jenny, registered with me. Jenny was in her early thirties and had recently moved back into town after splitting up with her partner. Jenny's case was slightly unusual: she had developed a benign, slow-growing brain tumor two years earlier and, with it, epilepsy. She was taking several anticonvulsant drugs on repeat prescription. I spoke to Jenny on the telephone and asked her to come in to the office to meet me and review her case.

"No," she said adamantly. She did not want to come in, she said. Why should she? She was already under the neurologist team. She just wanted her prescription. Her notes confirmed her history, and so we settled into an uncomfortable stand off. I would prescribe her medication without meeting her in person.

This went on until last year when the social worker who was involved with Jenny called me. Did I know Jenny was now confined to bed? Did I know Jenny's mother had been sending the home health assistants away nearly every visit?

No, I didn't. In fact, I did not even know Jenny had a social worker.

The social worker explained that Jenny's mother had become very protective of her daughter and was providing all her care herself. She was cancelling any prearranged visits by health or social care workers. In England we make house calls, and I decided to visit Jenny and her family unannounced.

Jenny lived in a small two-bedroom house on a council housing estate in the western suburbs. Her parents, with a traditional working-class respect for the family doctor, welcomed me in and took me to Jenny's bedroom. There lay Jenny. Bedridden for the last six months as her tumor had slowly grown and completed her left-side paralysis. She was confined to a single room by the misguided protective instinct of her mother and her (smothering) love.

Jenny's mother was anxious to impress on me that Jenny could not go on like this. I agreed. She had read that the local authority would provide, free of charge, adaptions and room additions to the home for deserving cases. It was quite clear that she felt Jenny was a deserving case and she wanted her free addition.

I was not sure that was the next step. It was difficult to judge whether her mother's motivation was to improve quality of life for Jenny or get as much as possible from "the system." Jenny's case alarmed me, so I called a case conference at my office to which all involved health and social care workers were invited.

At the meeting, the social worker said she was worried that Jenny was a vulnerable adult and it was unclear whether her mother was acting in Jenny's best interests. When Jenny's mother cancelled the visits of the caregivers, was this Jenny's wish or her mothers? They would often be told that Jenny did not want to see them today, but they would not be allowed to see Jenny to confirm this.

The social worker was concerned about the fact that Jenny's mother was providing all the care herself. This was effectively confining Jenny to bed and could be interpreted as a form of abuse. It was unclear whether her mother's overprotection was malicious or misguided. The social worker decided to call on Jenny to explore her wishes and her capacity to make decisions and to better understand her mother's perspective.

The neurology nurse specialist suggested visiting Jenny with the occupational therapist and physiotherapist to assess Jenny's physical capability. Because Jenny's mother was so keen on her free house addition, making an assessment of need was seen as part of that process.

Over the coming days, the social worker visited and found that Jenny did indeed have the capacity to make her own decisions but was fearful of her future. She had avoided having brain scans for two years as she was scared of what they might show. Jenny's mother had become mistrustful of caregivers who sometimes failed to appear, were often different individuals, and who, she felt, could not provide the loving care she wanted for her daughter.

The nurse specialist and the therapist found that Jenny was able to sit and could be transferred out of bed into a chair, despite her one-sided paralysis. She did seem excessively drowsy. I visited her at home to reassess her medication and take blood tests to monitor her anticonvulsant levels.

Jenny expressed a wish to have an up-to-date brain scan.

At the next meeting in my office the team decided to offer Jenny a five-day stay at the inpatient neurology rehabilitation unit. This would allow the rehabilitation therapists to fully assess Jenny's physical and neurological abilities and communicate with her about her wishes and concerns away from her mother while the brain scan was undertaken.

The head of the home care agency attended the meeting and discussed the ongoing difficulty that Jenny's mother was not permitting caregivers to actually care for her daughter. She managed to arrange consistent caregivers to ensure continuity of personnel for Jenny. I visited Jenny's mother with the nurse specialist to explain that Jenny had expressed a wish to determine the care she received. We arranged for Jenny to have a telephone at her bedside so she could be contacted when necessary. Subsequently, Jenny was asked via telephone whether she wished to cancel care, and the access to her by caregivers improved.

The blood tests showed the anticonvulsant levels were above the therapeutic range. Unfortunately, lowering the dose made Jenny more wakeful and restless. She started hallucinating about strangers living in the attic of the house. I called the rehabilitation consultant, and we arranged to visit Jenny at home together. Jenny and her mother were distressed by her hallucinations and were keen for her to take a small dose of antipsychotic that was suggested. The hallucinations resolved.

The following week Jenny was admitted for her rehabilitation assessment and had a brain scan showing slow progress of the tumor over the previous two years without involvement of new tissues. It did, however, remain inoperable.

Being out of her bedroom for the first time in nearly a year gave Jenny a new outlook. She gained trust in the team around her, and her mother started to relinquish some of her caretaking duties and spend more time on her relationship with her daughter.

Jenny's mother's house has still not had an addition. Jenny still has a dense paralysis and a brain tumor. She is, however, being cared for more appropriately, and the individuals on the team working with her are communicating with her and her mother. Everyone has a greater understanding of her or his role, and Jenny is no longer bedridden or confined to her room.

This outcome was a direct result of a number of face-to-face conversations with multiple health and social care workers. If I had continued to rely on communication via notes in a chart or a computerized medical record, Jenny would have continued to deteriorate and her mother would have put the barriers up even higher. We would never have gotten close to Jenny. It was only when someone directly contacted me and relayed her concerns that things began to change for all of us. These conversations with various care workers helped me to understand the variety of skills and services that were available; I didn't shoulder this entire burden on my own. Because we all engaged in a series of conversations—with the kind of actual give-and-take real conservations produce—in which someone would make a suggestion and someone else might agree or disagree, finally robust solutions would emerge that gained the ownership of the wider team. In this way, we were able to break down the shell of confusion, negative assumptions, and differences to find out what this disempowered patient really wanted.

• • •

MARTYN DIAPER, MD is a family doctor in Winchester, England. He is Clinical Lead for Safer Care for the National Health Service (NHS) Improving Quality Delivery Team, Chairman of NHS England's Patient Safety Expert Group for Primary Care, and Clinical Director for Integrated Community Services in South East Hampshire.

The Telephone Call

Karen Gold

I am the social worker on a team of nurses, physicians, technicians, and administrative and intake staff at a sexual health clinic in Toronto. Many of the patients are young and careening through unplanned pregnancies, relationship problems, family instability, and dating violence. Many carry the scars of traumatic loss or abuse. The emotional distress clients bring to the clinic can overshadow their medical needs. In the swamp of everyday practice, emotional distresses spill over the edges of clinical encounters, making our brief interactions with patients more challenging as we are forced to acknowledge that their lives are more complicated than we are prepared or trained to handle.

Working at the clinic is also a study in uncertainty, as we never know where conversations with clients will go. We try to piece together stories from the fragments clients give us, what they tell us (and what they don't), and the information gleaned from the medical chart. These narratives are not always straightforward.

This was true of a certain phone conversation a nurse had with a patient. As I arrived at the clinic one day, the nurse greeted me with a chart in her hand. "This young woman came in last week. She has some medical complications that we're dealing with, but she didn't sound too good when I called her yesterday. Maybe you could give her a call?" I hesitated for a moment, not sure how to respond, and I realized I had a choice to make. The patient had not said anything explicitly about needing urgent help, and there was no sign of obvious risk or immediate harm. Did I want to call her and chance opening up emotional wounds that perhaps should stay closed? I have learned the hard way that well-intentioned (but misplaced) interventions can do more harm than good.

But there was something in the nurse's voice that made me stop and consider her request. She continued, "She's kind of hard to understand because she's got a quiet voice, but you can tell she's really having a hard time." Although I considered saying, "It doesn't sound urgent" or "I've got a packed schedule and don't think I'll have time today," I was well aware that experienced clinicians pick up on subtle cues when something isn't quite right. Call it intuition, a gut sense, practice wisdom, or pattern recognition, I have learned it is often valuable knowledge and not to be dismissed.

I was also conscious that how I chose to respond in that moment would contribute to the tenor of our relationship as colleagues. Collaboration between physicians and nurses has (rightly) been the focus of much interprofessional attention, as their ability to work together respectfully and productively shapes the kind of care patients receive in acute and inpatient settings. But the relationship between nurses and social workers, so often pivotal in outpatient and mental health settings, has received limited attention. It is a curious omission, given our overlapping roles in addressing psychosocial concerns and the need to work closely to respond to clients' emotional needs. Mutual respect and flexibility are keys to good working relationships.

So I agreed to call, knowing that both of us would feel better if I checked in with this client. I went down the hall to the counseling office where I could get some privacy and quiet. I quickly flipped through the pages of the thick chart, glancing at the last entry made by the nurse with whom I had just spoken, and dialed the client's phone number. Anticipating a recorded voice message, I was surprised when a young woman answered the phone.

After verifying that it was the patient, I began by saying, "Hi, my name is Karen Gold and I am a social worker at the clinic. You saw the nurse here the other day, and we just want to check in and see how you are doing." I was half expecting (and hoping) to hear, "I'm fine. Thank you for calling," so I could continue with my scheduled appointments. I was already starting to think about my other cases and patients waiting to be seen. Instead, the young woman with the quiet voice said, "Not so good. I want to kill myself."

I froze, letting her words sink in while at the same time searching for a way to respond. Struggling to think of a way to keep the conversation going, I asked her to tell me more about what was going on. As she began to talk, I began to formulate a safety plan. She mentioned her father, and I wondered whether he might play a role. I wanted to keep her talking until I had assurance (or a promise) that she would be okay.

I finally ended the call when she agreed to phone her father and make arrangements to go to the nearby hospital. Satisfied that a plan was in place and that the client knew she could call back if she needed to, I said goodbye.

For a long moment after hanging up, fragments of the conversation swirled through my mind. I felt unsure how to document what had happened in the sparse language of the chart. I wondered how I could capture the conversation so that the next practitioner who saw her understood the severity of her distress and the crisis unfolding in her life. I wrote a brief summary, trying to translate her words and my concerns into professional shorthand. I couldn't shake the feeling that despite having charted the latest development, I needed to do more.

I surfaced from the now-silent office, chart in hand, and headed back to the nurses' station. I was relieved to see the nurse who approached me with the chart, and I sat down beside her. Beginning with "It's good that I called. Your instincts were right," I told her what happened. We talked for a few minutes about the woman with the quiet voice, both of us hoping she would make it through this difficult time. I made a mental note to call the client back in a few days and check in with her.

At work, later that evening, I still had the young woman on my mind as I reflected on how a seemingly simple phone call could take a serious turn. I thought about the nurse, now busy with another patient in another part of the clinic. I was glad we had that brief conversation when I arrived at the clinic and that I listened to her intuition. It led to another unexpected—but vital—conversation that may have saved a life.

. . .

KAREN GOLD, ITDK has been a Social Worker and Educator in health care for over twenty years. She coordinates a hospital-based interprofessional education program and is currently working on a PhD on narrative reflective writing by health care practitioners.

Interprofessional Learners Sharing Our Stories

Mandy Lowe, Tracy Paulenko, and Lynne Sinclair

In health care, interprofessional education (IPE) is often conceived of as something designed primarily to instruct students as future health care professionals. While successful IPE programs certainly have an influence on students, they can also have a broader impact—influencing the educators who teach students to become future professionals, the staff these professionals will work with, and of course the patients whose care they provide. Rather than reinforcing traditional siloed education and practice, IPE programs designed for students can create the broader context in which interprofessional practice becomes a reality. Through IPE, we can learn not only about what students need to know to practice interprofessionally but also about the skills faculty and staff need to master and practice in order to make ongoing IPE and interprofessional care (IPC) a reality.

The three of us had been involved in interprofessional education and care for many years when we worked together at the Toronto Rehabilitation Institute (Toronto Rehab), University Health Network. Toronto Rehab has long pioneered IPE/IPC for both students and clinicians. When the governments of both Canada and the province of Ontario mandated and began to finance IPE/IPC in the mid-2000s, our past education and practice were given a tremendous boost.

In an effort to pave the way for interprofessional education at the clinical level, in 2004 the Toronto Rehab piloted a structured IPE placement in which a team of students from different professions was placed in the same practice setting at the same time. Students were supported by clinical facilitators who had received interprofessional faculty development (education for the educators) and who worked for either the direct clinical unit or the broader organization. We had learned that just because someone is a skilled facilitator or mentor in a particular field (e.g., their own profession) it does not necessarily mean that that person can teach at a highly skilled interprofessional level. Our facilitators need to be prepared to mentor and facilitate interprofessionally so that students can learn about, from, and with one another to improve interprofessional collaboration and care.

This model of interprofessional learning was inspired by rural health care placement programs in New Mexico and Northern Ontario and was the first of its kind in Toronto. Since then, use of this approach to enable interprofessional learning in practice settings has grown significantly with the development of a toolkit that is available for anyone to use (www.ipe.utoronto.ca). This work has had tremendous influence not only on student learning but has positively affected both the work of health care providers in the hospital and in overall direct patient care. We have each written a story that illustrates the kind of positive synergies that emerge from this model of student learning. In these stories we see examples of how teamwork and interprofessional collaboration have an impact on educators, staff, and ultimately on patients under their care.

EDUCATING THE EDUCATORS

By Mandy Lowe

I have shared this story about student learning and my own interprofessional facilitation skills on several occasions. It demonstrates how critical it is for those of us who are teachers, facilitators, or mentors to be acutely aware of our own professional lens in interprofessional learning. At the time of this story, I had worked clinically for many years as an occupational therapist in a rehabilitation setting. I was also a clinical educator in occupational therapy, a leadership role within the hospital that supported occupational therapists in their ongoing professional development while working to enable student learning. I had the privilege of working with some exceptionally collaborative interprofessional teams and hoped that my contribution as a facilitator of interprofessional learning in an IPE placement would enable rich learning for the students.

I was partnered with a colleague from physiotherapy (my cofacilitator), and we led a group of eight students from a range of professions in weekly interprofessional tutorials through the placement.

On one occasion, the students said that they wanted to learn more about "transfers," a learning objective we were confident we could help them meet. We quickly scheduled some critical learning opportunities for the session; we brought in a range of transfer devices and wheelchairs and invited a colleague to share information about how to work with them with the students. The students were engaged and appreciative throughout the session. At the end of the session, a pharmacy student approached me and told me how much she enjoyed the session. I will forever be grateful for what she said next. She told me that the session—interesting though it was—had also surprised her. "Why?" I asked. She replied that she had anticipated the session would focus on processes associated with transferring patients from acute care to inpatient rehabilitation, not physically transferring patients from a bed to a wheelchair.

Now it was my turn to be surprised. And it was my turn to learn! It had simply not occurred to me that in planning and giving the session I was viewing "transfers" exclusively through my own professional lens. As an occupational therapist, transfers have a particular significance and meaning. Say the word "transfer" to an OT or PT, and he or she will likely think about the skills and equipment needed to move a patient from bed to wheelchair, from the wheelchair to the bathtub, and so on. Transfers are also important to many of us because they are part of the crucial process of enabling clients to become more independent. Because of this, we enthusiastically planned this session around our own shared understanding of transfers. What I realized after this encounter was that, in my enthusiasm, I had assumed everyone was on the same page, and thus I had missed the opportunity to stop and clarify the meaning of transfers in different professions. Since that time, I have learned to become much more aware of differences in meanings and jargon used; I strive to seek opportunities for clarification across professions, whether in my own work with students, staff, or as part of faculty development. In essence, I gained a firsthand appreciation of the unique skills required to be a truly effective facilitator of interprofessional education.

· · ·

MANDY LOWE, OT is Director of Education and Professional Development, University Health Network, University of Toronto. She is also

Associate Director, Centre for Interprofessional Education, University of Toronto and Assistant Professor, Department of Occupational Science and Occupational Therapy, Faculty of Medicine, University of Toronto.

IMPACT ON STAFF COLLABORATION

By Tracy Paulenko

As an IPE leader, I have the privilege of seeing numerous IPE student groups present what they learn when they are introduced to inter-professional care in the clinical setting. A particularly salient presentation was by an IPE student group on our neurological inpatient rehabilitation unit regarding weekend passes. In rehabilitation, it is essential for health care teams to provide patients with opportunities to try their new skills in safe, supportive environments. Weekend passes afford such opportunities in which patients spend time in their own home prior to discharge.

Weekends home require high levels of collaboration and communication among the different health care providers involved. Typically, social workers, speech-language pathologists, physical therapists, pharmacists, occupational therapists, nurses, and doctors are involved in this process. These team members must ensure that patients and family members have the proper education, skills, and resources for a safe, optimal experience. On return to the rehabilitation unit, these same team members, together with the patient and family, assess what went well and determine what to do differently the next time to safely meet the patient's and family's goals for discharge.

This particular IPE student group presented on the interprofessional health care team's current processes and resources for weekend passes. They identified general areas of need through patients' and families' post–weekend pass discussions, as well as lessons learned from the teamwork literature. The postpresentation discussion among the IP health care team and students was open and insightful—it was the impetus for the team to take action. Led by their advanced-practice leader, the team embarked on a project to optimize weekend passes. To determine the gaps, they further examined their processes and documentation, held a focus group for patients and families, performed a limited environmental scan, and reviewed the literature.

They discovered that patients and families found the weekend pass process fragmented and confusing, given that each health care provider would instruct them through their own professional lens about what to do and not to do while on weekend pass. This could mean up to half a dozen professional encounters for the patient and family on the afternoon before a weekend home, with individual team members bearing either the same or potentially contradictory information. The team quickly realized they needed a collaborative approach to redesign the process and create an interprofessional documentation tool.

Subsequently, for each weekend pass, nursing, occupational therapy, and physical therapy work together to create the patient and family instructions, with input from other relevant team members. These instructions are based on functional activities of everyday life that the patient will need to do when at home; for example, bathing, dressing, eating, sleeping, and socializing with family and friends. These weekend pass instructions are now succinctly written on a short interprofessional documentation form and are reviewed with the patient and family by a team member prior to the weekend pass. It has improved the weekend pass process so well from the perspectives of both the team members and patients and their families that other interprofessional care units are considering using it to optimize their patients' rehabilitation planning in preparation for discharge. Who could have imagined that a structured IPE student clinical placement group's exploration of the teamwork involved in weekend passes would have such broad implications for the health care staff?

· · ·

TRACY PAULENKO, PT is an Interprofessional Education/Care and Professional Development Leader, Toronto Rehabilitation Institute, University Health Network and an Instructor in the Department of Physical Therapy, Faculty of Medicine, University of Toronto.

IMPACT ON DIRECT PATIENT CARE

By Lynne Sinclair

The student discussions in tutorials that occur in IPE are not just an academic exercise. The goal of interprofessional education is the kind of interprofessional practice that can have a profound impact on direct patient care. I was an interprofessional facilitator for a group of six students who were on a geriatric day hospital IPE student placement. The students had been meeting weekly for patient-themed tutorials in which they discussed topics of care related to the patients that they shared on the unit. As she was talking with the other students, the speech-language pathology (SLP) student explained that she was encountering several challenges in her treatment sessions with a patient who was presenting with swallowing difficulties. This patient was short of breath and very fatigued and thus was finding it too difficult to work on his speech in his therapy sessions.

The students listened quietly, and as the facilitator I tried to encourage the others to ask questions and learn more about the treatments that SLPs can provide. An occupational therapy student raised her hand. She told the group that, with her supervisor, she had just worked with the same patient and they had made some seating changes to the patient's wheelchair. These changes to the cushion and the back support enabled the patient to sit in a more upright position and to extend his back to a more functional posture. I watched with awe as the face of the SLP student lit up with excitement. She asked if this might help the patient to swallow and breathe easier. The SLP student exclaimed that she had no idea that OTs helped with seating posture.

In the group, we talked about why a seating posture can affect a patient's ability to take a full breath, swallow, and speak and therefore to have more energy for therapy. One by one the students appeared to fully realize the impact that shared communication and knowledge of one another's roles can have on direct patient care. I have often thought back to this occasion and am reminded each time that teamwork is a critical factor in determining the effectiveness of patient care. On the conclusion of IPE placements, students reflect on and evaluate these experiences and often say they will have a profound effect on their practice as they know more about roles and resources on the health care team.

Each of us has frequently experienced that IPE is not an end point but provides an opening to have an impact not only on the students but those of us who teach them, those staff members who can either reinforce the traditional hidden curricula of health care training or model new and more productive team attitudes, behavior, and practice. Ultimately, the true test of IPE is how it affects practice and thus the kind of care our patients receive. This positive circle of continuous learning and synergy of working together as a team has the potential to create a transformative change in the way we practice health care.

· · ·

LYNNE SINCLAIR, PT is an Education Consultant and Innovative Program and External Development Lead, Centre for Interprofessional Education, University of Toronto. She is also Assistant Professor, Department of Physical Therapy, Faculty of Medicine, University of Toronto.

Part 2

THE DANGERS AND DAMAGE OF POOR TEAMWORK

The kind of poor practice described in this part is, sadly, all too common in the contemporary health care system. Poor work relationships and lack of teamwork don't only result in tears or hurt feelings. Lack of teamwork causes actual harm and even death to patients. Although we worry most about harm to patients, they are not the only ones who experience the downstream impact of the failure to teach people who work in health care the necessary skills to work on teams. Those who work in the health care system at every level are also the victims of poor teamwork. They often experience physical and emotional problems when teamwork is the exception rather than the rule and lack of respect, the ecological norm.[1]

In the absence of collaborative work, patient harm may result from many factors. Because of the stress created by disrespectful or abusive behavior, health care workers, on whose judgment and attentiveness patients depend, have a very difficult time returning to their activities after they have experienced such behavior.[2] Many health care managers believe that health care workers can somehow overcome negative experiences because they are "professionals." According to this myth, their "professionalism" will magically override any response that the brain triggers when confronted with stressful conditions. Neuroscientists and cognitive psychologists are increasingly documenting that this belief is fiction, not fact. When a physician yells at a nurse, or a nurse at an aide, the HPA response is set in motion, and without serious and systematic training in dealing with conflict, the chemical cascade that results is difficult to interrupt.

The stress response may make it physiologically difficult—if not, at times, impossible—for people to return to their work caring for patients in a way that allows the mobilization of their full attention to the tasks at hand. Anyone who has responded to a cardiac arrest or serious deterioration of a patient understands the power of the fight-or-flight response. Even when the patient has been stabilized, the chemicals unleashed course through the caregiver's body, and it may take hours for the person to fully unwind. The same thing happens when people are on the receiving end of abusive, uncivil comments that dismiss their concerns, denigrate their knowledge and skill, and fail to acknowledge their stake and commitment to their work, in particular, and patient care, in general.

Even when people are able to return to work, the result of the kinds of behaviors described in part 2 function as a relational nocebo effect that may prevent them from being able to provide optimum patient care or work relationships. Disrespectful or abusive behaviors have a negative impact even when the cast of characters changes and an abusive colleague or co-worker is no longer present. At best, people socialized in antiteam environments may end up being task focused or see only their own piece of the patient care process. No one really knows who "owns the patient." Nor do they know whom to go to for assistance in a timely manner. With no clear, collaboratively created plan, people lack a broad perspective, which, in turn, makes it easier for patients to fall through the cracks because obvious signs of deterioration may be missed.[3]

As we have said, Hackman's definition of good teamwork involves the ability of teams to work together over and over again. Just as a good team learns the lessons of excellent practice, lack of teamwork deskills. Poor practice in the area of teamwork leads to the opposite of what Captain Sullenberger describes in the introduction to part 1. As countless reports of tragic accidents highlight, when there is poor leadership and unassertive team membership, groups of people who need to become hyperorganized in a crisis instead become disorganized.[4]

When poor practice is the deviance that is normalized in health care, those who work in this closed system become fearful of change as well as of one another.[5] Research on how the brain works that has focused on what is called "negativity bias" helps us understand that people who are subject to abusive, disrespectful behavior are seriously affected by it. This is because the brain registers negative experiences far more strongly than positive ones.[6] (Think about it, you have a great day and then a fight with a friend, colleague, partner, spouse, and your day—and night—are ruined.) This means that a nurse who has been yelled at by one surgeon will probably not be able to return to tasks with optimum attention and may also begin to assume that surgeons in general don't listen and respond to legitimate concerns because they see them as challenges to their authority. If excessive workload and task saturation are added to behavioral problems, we have a perfect patient safety storm.[7] If encounters are positive and respectful, people will build on this foundation going forward. If they are unpleasant and disrespectful, they will certainly not look forward to the next time they have to work together. Because our brains register negative experiences far more forcefully than positive ones, this negativity bias becomes hard to overcome and can contaminate an entire unit or even institution. Neuroscientists are helping us understand just why one rotten apple can spoil the barrel and just why—and how—the people we interact with today will have a huge influence on how we work together tomorrow.

In health care today, several medical errors and injuries, such as central line–associated blood stream infections (CLABSI) or leaving surgical instruments inside a patient, have been declared to be "never events." These are "adverse events that are serious, largely preventable, and of concern to both the public and health care providers for the purpose of public accountability."[8] Given the lapses in teamwork described in these stories, it becomes clear why so many "never events" seem to be so ever present. To eliminate them, perhaps we need a new category of "never events" that applies to teamwork and communication among those who work in health care. Things such as

- never refuse to help a teammate;
- never refuse to come to the bedside to assess a patient when requested;
- never—ever—humiliate anyone with whom you work;
- never yell at someone lower on the health care ladder;
- never deny you did it when you did do it; and
- never . . . (fill in the blank).

I Had to Yell at the Nurse

Charles Bardes

"I had to yell at the nurse." The speaker is a young doctor, Mark. The scene is morning report, a daily conference in which resident physicians discuss their cases with the chief of medicine. On the previous evening, Mark had admitted a patient whose blood tests showed a perilously low level of sodium. His job had been to analyze the problem, fix it, and tell the story to the group.

"And why did you have to yell at the nurse?" asks a visitor, a physician.

"Well, I thought at first that she must have made a mistake. You never see a sodium that low unless someone has drawn blood above an IV line or something dumb like that."

"What did you do?"

"I rechecked the blood test myself and sent it stat. The repeat value was the same. So it wasn't a mistake."

"Why do you think you yelled at the nurse?"

"Well, I guess I shouldn't have done that. I was worried. The patient could have had a seizure with a sodium that low."

"Were you scared, maybe?"

"Maybe I was. I'd actually never seen a sodium that low. That's why I thought it must have been a mistake. I wasn't sure what to do."

"So that's why you yelled?"

"Yeah, I guess so."

"So why did you yell at the nurse?"

"Who else could have made the mistake? The blood test machine? Who else was there to yell at?"

"Maybe at the chief of medicine, sitting next to me here, for putting you in a life-threatening situation when you didn't know quite what to do?"

The chief shifts uncomfortably in his chair.

"I don't think so!"

The chief chuckles a little.

"And did you apologize to the nurse?"

"Well, no."

"Should you?"

"Yeah, I guess so."

The chief speaks up. "All right, enough of the nurse. Why do you think the sodium was so low?"

· · ·

CHARLES BARDES, MD is Professor of Clinical Medicine and Associate Dean at Weill Cornell Medical College, where he practices and teaches internal medicine. His books include *Essential Skills in Internal Medicine*, a guide for students and interns, and *Pale Faces: The Masks of Anemia*, a cultural history of anemia. His essays and articles have appeared in medical journals, including the *New England Journal of Medicine, Medical Education, Academic Medicine,* and *Teaching and Learning in Medicine,* the literary journals *Agni* and *Literary Imagination,* and the anthology *Becoming a Doctor.*

Lack of Teamwork Further Complicates a Case

Ramon Berguer

CASE DESCRIPTION

A fifty-six-year-old man with a history of intravenous drug abuse (used heroin the day before admission), hepatitis C, diabetes mellitus type 2, smoking, and morbid obesity presented to the Emergency Department with nausea, vomiting, and right upper quadrant abdominal pain for the past twenty-four hours. His physical exam demonstrated slight jaundice as well as tenderness on palpation in the right upper quadrant of the abdomen. His laboratory studies revealed a slightly elevated serum bilirubin, which could suggest a problem with the liver, gallbladder, or bile ducts. He also had a low-grade temperature of 100.3. The alkaline phosphatase level was slightly elevated, and liver enzymes were near 1000, also indicating a potential problem with liver, gallbladder, or bile ducts. An ultrasound of the abdomen showed a contracted gallbladder and multiple gallstones. A diagnosis of acute cholecystitis (inflammation of the gallbladder) was made, and a surgical consultation was obtained.

The surgeon on call saw the patient the next morning and thought that, due to the elevated liver enzymes and bilirubin, the patient might also have cholangitis, an inflammation/infection of the bile ducts. The patient was taken to surgery on the same day and underwent a laparoscopic removal of the gallbladder as well as a cholangiogram, a dye picture of the bile ducts. The gallbladder was found to have severe wall thickening and multiple adhesions around it, indicating a chronic inflammatory process. The intraoperative cholangiogram was normal.

Following surgery the patient initially improved, but then he began to complain of increasingly severe abdominal pain and distention, and his liver enzyme levels increased even further. The hospitalist team contacted the surgeon who was off-site. Due to the increased liver enzyme levels, and therefore suspicion of a problem in the bile ducts or the duct from the pancreas, he suggested a gastroenterology (GI) consultation for a possible endoscopic retrograde cholangiopancreatography (ERCP). This involves passing an endoscope into the stomach and then the small intestine and subsequently putting a small catheter through the endoscope into the pancreatic and bile ducts as they empty into the intestine.

The GI consultant spoke to the hospitalist team by phone and initially thought that the patient had acute hepatitis, probably from drug use and that treatment should be supportive care. As the patient's condition worsened, the treating team continued to consult with the gastroenterologist. The patient's condition worsened and rapidly deteriorated, and he was transferred to the intensive care unit. On the sixth day after surgery an internal medicine consult was obtained. One suggestion was to perform a paracentesis (sticking a small catheter into the abdominal cavity) to check for blood or infection in the abdomen. As the team prepared to perform the procedure, the patient had a sudden cardiac arrest and, despite resuscitation efforts, died. A limited postmortem exam was performed and revealed some blood-tinged fluid in the abdominal cavity, a healing surgical site without complications, and mild liver inflammation. No clear cause for his cardiac arrest was established.

STRUCTURE OF CARE

Care at this Safety Net facility (a public hospital whose patient population includes many people on Medicaid or who are uninsured), is delivered with a system of family medicine (FM) hospitalists who work with medical and surgical specialists. Patients with possible surgical problems are admitted to the inpatient family medicine service by the hospitalist team. After initial evaluation, the surgeon is contacted if a consultation is needed. Operative care is provided primarily by surgeons, and postoperative care is supervised directly by the FM hospitalist and resident with the surgeon providing input based on the specific needs of each patient. Surgeons meet with the FM hospitalists at monthly peer review meetings and administratively several times a year to discuss system issues. Medical specialty consultations are available, but staffing is somewhat limited.

SURGEON'S POINT OF VIEW

This was a heavyset and friendly patient who had severe and recurrent abdominal pain in his right upper quadrant. He admitted to a history of drug abuse and a history of hepatitis but said he was currently clean. His abdominal ultrasound showed he had gallstones, and he had some inflammation, evidenced by elevated liver-function tests. His pain was consistent with classic biliary colic (pain in the right upper quadrant of the abdomen due to gallstones). I had recommended a laparoscopic cholecystectomy, which he underwent the next morning. The case was difficult, in part because of the problem of separating the gallbladder from surrounding structures. Sometimes these difficulties are so serious that we have to convert to a traditional open operation, but that was not necessary in this case, which was conducted completely laparoscopically without an injury to any adjacent structures. After surgery, the patient stated that his pain was gone.

I assumed he did well and that he had been discharged. About four days later, I was called and told he was having some medical issues slowing his recovery and discharge. I was told that he had had an "ileus" (i.e., his bowel stopped working) and perhaps full-blown hepatitis, and some fluid and breathing problems, and that the GI service had been consulted by phone. I was called a couple of days later and informed that he had died. After overcoming my astonishment, I asked what had happened and what problems had developed, and whether anyone with surgical experience had been asked to come back and evaluate the patient. The resident and hospitalist FP had pretty much handled his increasing problems without raising red flags to let us know his recovery was not as anticipated.

FM HOSPITALIST'S POINT OF VIEW

I first met the patient two days after he had had a laparoscopic cholecystectomy for middle upper abdomen and right upper quadrant pain with abnormal liver-function tests. When I was working with the resident that morning, she and I noticed that the liver enzymes and function tests had worsened despite the surgery. The resident called the surgeon who had operated, and he recommended that we call the on-call gastroenterologist as there were no further surgical interventions warranted. The concern at this time was for an acute hepatitis or an impacted common bile duct stone, two problems that are managed very differently. The gastroenterologist spoke at length to the resident, while I sat next to her. The gastroenterologist had very strong opinions that the patient was mismanaged by having his gallbladder removed and that the patient really had a drug-induced acute hepatitis, despite a normal urine toxicology screen on admission for illicit drugs. He recommended supportive care for the patient's acute hepatitis. I went to examine and speak to the patient and noted that he had a round distended abdomen, and he said that it was a little bigger than usual. He also denied that he had used any illicit substances recently.

On the next day the liver tests started to show some improvement, but the patient started to complain of increased abdominal distension. His low blood level of sodium had worsened, and he had an elevated white blood count of 15,000, which indicated some inflammation or infection. The resident contacted the same gastroenterologist while I sat next to her. He recommended continued supportive care and stopping the patient's antibiotics. This was surely because he didn't think the patient had a bacterial infection and one doesn't treat drug-induced hepatitis with an antibiotic. I again examined the patient and took his vital signs, which were stable, and he had no fever. Despite some increased abdominal distension there were no signs on exam of an intra-abdominal surgical complication.

On the second day that I saw this patient the liver tests continued to slowly improve, but the white blood count increased to 25,000, while a urine culture grew *Staphylococcus aureus*, and his sodium level continued to be low. The resident again contacted the gastroenterologist, and he repeated his recommendation of supportive care. He had not seen the patient or written any recommendations in the chart up to this time. The patient continued to complain of abdominal discomfort, and he appeared more distended, but again, when we examined him, he had no signs of the kind of sensitivity that would suggest the urgent need for surgical intervention. He was started on antibiotics for a urinary tract infection, and we decided to give him some intravenous fluids for his low sodium levels. That same evening he developed shortness of breath and needed oxygen and was transferred to the intermediate care unit. Despite these changes, his blood pressure and heart rate remained stable.

The following morning he had further increased abdominal distension, but he had received four liters of fluid in an attempt to treat the low sodium. His white blood count increased to 65,000, but he remained with stable blood pressure, heart rate, and no fever. With such a high white blood cell count, we were concerned that he had a systemic bacterial infection, and so we added more aggressive antibiotics to the treatment. Given the dramatic elevation in his white blood cell count, we also considered a possible lab error and had his blood count done again. The gastroenterologist was again contacted, and, in spite of all this, he made no further changes in his recommendations. I was frustrated that I was not getting the help that I needed and went to discuss the patient with one of my mentors at this hospital. This person suggested getting an internal medicine consultation to get another set of eyes on the patient and to see where I may have missed something. Around the time that the medicine consultant began to review the patient's chart, the repeat complete blood cell blood returned demonstrating a low hemoglobin (6.5) and an even higher white blood cell count of 72,000. A blood transfusion and fluids were ordered. As the resident and medicine consultant were getting ready to perform a diagnostic paracentesis to sample the fluid in the abdomen for infection, the patient suddenly became unresponsive and died soon thereafter, despite attempts at resuscitation. The cause of death remains unknown even after a limited autopsy.

I contacted the general surgeon the following day to let him know that the patient had died. We discussed some of the details of the case. He was not accusatory or judgmental about the care provided and did ask if someone from the surgery department had been contacted. I replied that I had not called a surgeon that morning to see the patient because I did not believe he had a surgical problem.

I was contacted two months later by the gastroenterologist, who told me in a very authoritative manner that I had grossly mismanaged the patient and that I was responsible for the patient's death. He said I had not followed his directions and recommendations and I was an incompetent physician. Prior to calling me, this gastroenterologist had been discussing the details of this patient's case with other physicians at the hospital who were not involved in the patient's care and also telling them that I was incompetent and was responsible for this patient's death. These doctors, who knew very little about the details of the patient's case, would approach me and say that the gastroenterologist told them about the case and then shake their head in disbelief. I felt as though my name and abilities as a physician were being slandered, and I felt ashamed to show up at work every day. At the same time, I felt angry that the doctor who was supposed to be helping me manage the patient was putting all the blame on my shoulders and not accepting any responsibility for his own role in the patient's care. The doctors who had actually reviewed the case and knew the details and complexities were supportive and understanding.

My resident and I had had extensive conversations about this patient. We had spent considerable time each day discussing him on rounds, and we made a point each day to see him at the bedside together, something we don't always do. We both felt frustrated that the gastroenterologist would spend so much time on the phone but had not been to see the patient once. There were no clear management recommendations other than supportive care, and neither I nor the resident had the understanding that he wanted us to have further imaging done on the patient. Although the gastroenterologist had a role in the care of the patient, it was very important to me as the hospitalist that I should take all responsibility for the patient's care and subsequent death as I was the attending physician and mentor for the resident.

GASTROENTEROLOGIST'S POINT OF VIEW

The gastroenterology service was contacted on a weekend by a first-year resident on the surgery service who was instructed to contact

GI regarding obtaining an ERCP on a complex case with underlying liver disease, substance use, and a presentation of acute cholecystitis. The on-call gastroenterologist reviewed the liver function tests and realized that they reflected an acute severe hepatitis, not common duct-stone disease, and advised against the study and suggested a workup for liver disease. The patient was taken to the operating room and the surgeon on call found severe cholecystitis and a normal biliary tree (i.e., the bile ducts were normal). I was contacted the following Monday by a third-year resident on the surgery/family practice service regarding the abnormal liver function tests, and I discussed possible etiologies and made recommendations for appropriate lab studies. Initially, the patient showed no signs of postoperative complications. The following day I was contacted by the same resident because the patient was complaining of distention of his abdomen, anorexia, and his white blood count had risen substantially. I made it clear to the resident that we were now dealing with a postoperative complication, not the liver issue, and outlined clearly a workup for postoperative distention of the abdomen to include abdominal x-rays followed by ultrasound of the abdomen if no bowel distention was seen. I reviewed the possible etiologies including ileus, obstruction, and fluid in the belly from bile leak or bleeding. I advised that the patient be seen by one of our attending surgeons if there was any abnormality. The third-year resident discussed these issues with her hospitalist attending who had seen the patient that day, but none of the suggested studies were ordered.

The following day I looked for the imaging results and contacted the same resident to see why they were not done. I got no clear answer and was told the patient was worse, with increasing distention and a white blood count that was now 30,000 and increased pain. I reviewed the recommended workup and advised her that an attending surgeon should see the patient that day and that they were certainly dealing with a major postoperative complication. Again, no such workup was done, nor was the patient seen by an on-site attending surgeon. The surgeon of record was off campus, and the resident contacted him by phone, and he relied on the information he was receiving from the hospitalist team. I am not aware of what suggestions, if any, he made, and he did not contact an on-site attending surgeon. The following day the patient was more critical. He was in the process of being moved to a critical care bed when he had a sudden arrest and could not be resuscitated. At postmortem he had about 2000 cc (two liters out of a blood volume of five liters) of bloody fluid in his abdomen but no obvious bleeding site. The gallbladder bed was noted to be normal for a postoperative cholecystectomy.

The issues in this case revolve around the phone communication between the GI service and the resident team not leading to appropriate action; that is, the absence of any attending surgical follow-up in a patient who clearly had a major complication from the surgery and was doing poorly. As the gastroenterologist, I might have contacted the hospitalist attending directly when the resident did not follow my initial recommendations, or I could have gone to the bedside and put a strong note in the chart, but I thought that since the patient was already on a surgical service with a postoperative problem that it could be handled by the surgeons present on that service. The failure of the family practice team to bring an on-site attending surgeon to the bedside is another major issue. It is not clear to me why that was so, but I conjecture that it's a common practice for postoperative care to be handled by the hospitalist attending and resident at our hospital, and they may have believed they were handling it appropriately. The lack of any direct involvement in postoperative care by the operating surgeon is yet another break in the chain of command that I think led to problems. In teaching institutions like ours there is often no continuous chain of ownership as there is in private practice, and in this case that proved to be very suboptimal.

QUALITY COORDINATOR'S POINT OF VIEW

The case was referred to the quality department as a postoperative mortality. As in other organizations, all mortalities are automatically reviewed, and most are cases in which everyone did their best and the systems worked well. I assumed this would be a case that would fall into that general category. But, very quickly, it became apparent that systems and processes did not work well, and old habits of practice had returned to create problems.

Peer review groups that reviewed the case all concluded that, although the eventual outcome might not have been prevented, there were some clear issues and possible system problems highlighted by it. They clearly identified that communication among providers may have been a barrier to effective, timely care. Although each isolated review group reached a similar conclusion, it does not allow for the intergroup communication needed to optimally "learn" from a case. So a multispecialty review was arranged, and all providers involved in the patient's care were assembled.

As the two primary attendings recounted the story of the patient, the atmosphere in the room became serious. These physicians were clearly reliving the experience, and it had obviously been a difficult one. Their emotions during this time were visible. They recounted a week of what I would describe as being alone in frustrating attempts to deal with the patient's clinic problems and input from multiple consultants. One GI medicine attending, whom they consulted, never wrote notes on his consults with them, so they were left with trying to remember their conversations with him as the patient's condition changed and they tried to adjust the treatment plan. Because this was a post-op mortality, the subject of surgery follow-up came up. This brought out very heated and passionate words from another hospitalist, who referred to a long past history of real or perceived grievances regarding teamwork and participation of surgery in patient care and coverage. Much of the meeting was spent "unpacking" the events and emotions around the incident and the impact of past events on them. Because of this, the meeting went past its allotted time.

MULTISPECIALTY REVIEW

This case was reviewed in both a peer review setting and in a multispecialty conference with all participants present. After charting the inpatient care and reviewing the records, it was concluded that despite the best efforts of the treating team, the patient had died of unexpected causes and that no clear mistake had been made. All the noted physiologic trends had been attended to and treated appropriately.

Specifically, it was unclear whether the patient had had hepatitis, and there appeared to be no surgical complication to explain the death. At the same time, all participants were unhappy about their experience in the care of this patient and felt that significant communication lapses had occurred that might have affected the care of this patient. There was also disagreement about the diagnosis of acute cholecystitis and whether the patient had needed surgery in the first place. Consultations with GI had been held by phone or in person, but the consultant did not see the patient or document the consultation. This led to disagreements about what the recommendations had actually been and when they were made. All participants felt the operating surgeon should have been involved in the postoperative care, but he was off-site and was not made aware of the deteriorating condition of the patient. Surgeons who were on-site during that time were not aware of the patient and were not consulted. The treating hospitalist and resident paid close attention to the patient's condition and worried about his deteriorating status. They thought they were dealing with a medical problem—acute hepatitis, based on the GI consultation—and thus they did not think they needed to contact a surgeon for help. The final recommendations were:

> 1. Surgeons or the on-call surgeon should be made aware of all postoperative problems in surgical patients.
> 2. Specialty-to-specialty communication should be direct and in person whenever possible to avoid "triangulation" with the treating hospitalist team.
> 3. Consultations should be documented in every case, and when needed the consultant should see the patient.

SIX-MONTH FOLLOW-UP

> 1. The registrars and surgeons have agreed that the operating surgeon or the surgeon on call that day must be called for any concerns or complications related to the procedure.
> 2. The GI service has been asked to document phone and in-person consultations in the medical record.

Communication is vital in any endeavor and no less so in health care. The postoperative recovery period is a fluid time during which circumstances change and complications may arise. It is critical that all the members of the health care team communicate properly, particularly making sure that the provider with the most knowledge and expertise in the situation be involved in the decision making at any time.

. . .

RAMON BERGUER, MD holds a bachelor's degree in computer science from the University of Michigan and completed his general surgery residency at the University of Colorado Health Sciences Center. He is currently a general surgeon at Contra Costa Regional Medical Center and John Muir Medical Center in the San Francisco Bay Area. He has published over fifty peer reviewed scientific papers as well as six book chapters in the areas of stress immunology, laparoscopic ergonomics, and the prevention of sharp injuries in the operating room. He is a consultant in surgical ergonomics and sharps injury prevention for medical device manufacturers.

Dying to Get to Baghdad

Peter Fish

When I was deployed to Iraq to work in a combat hospital, I was given many responsibilities. As medical officer-in-charge (OIC) of the hospital I was responsible for setting medical policy and operations and supervising medical officers. My job was complicated by the fact that I fulfilled these roles as a physician assistant—and thus was medically supervised by the physicians whom I administratively supervised—and by the fact that I was outranked by many of the medical providers whom I supervised.

As patient movement officer (PMO) my responsibility was to arrange for transportation of injured and ill patients to other medical facilities (usually by air) where they could obtain the care they needed. In a combat environment, this responsibility takes into consideration not only the medical condition of the patient but the safety of the flight crew as well. Patients whose medical conditions are not life threatening are held until the flying and combat conditions are less dangerous (because it's not worth possibly killing a four-person flight crew to confirm kidney stones with a CT scan). Those patients who are likely to die unless they are transferred to another facility are transported even if conditions are dangerous.

I also was the flight surgeon, responsible for supervising and guiding the flight medics who transported our patients.

These three roles were challenging enough individually, but one memorable evening their challenges converged.

Our hospital received an enemy prisoner of war who had been grievously wounded by other EPWs while he was in prison. The patient underwent damage-control surgery and was extremely unstable when he emerged from surgery. I was advised by medical staff (though not by the surgeon) as to his condition and the likelihood that he would die en route to the hospital in Baghdad. As PMO I passed the information along to the flight medics. Also as PMO,

I was reluctant to dispatch an aircrew to transfer a patient likely to die en route. As their flight surgeon, I advised the flight medics that if they thought that they were unable to safely care for this (or any patient) they were correct to refuse to accept the patient unless capable medical personnel accompanied him. It became apparent to me that the surgeon wanted the patient to die in the medevac helicopter (rather than our hospital) so that his surgical track record would not reflect the death of a patient under his care. Not only was this attempt to distance himself from the patient's death unethical, it would have put the careers of the flight medics in jeopardy, since their acceptance of the patient would have been questioned and they would have faced intense medical scrutiny.

The flight medics examined the patient, saw the situation and, recognizing that the intensive care equipment keeping him alive was beyond their level of training, refused to accept the patient into their care. The surgeon flew into a rage, confronted me accusing me of undermining his authority, insulted me in front of my staff, and, when I invited him to discuss the situation behind closed doors, physically assaulted me.

The medevac transfer was in fact undertaken when an ICU-trained nurse volunteered to accompany the patient. The patient did die en route. I pressed charges against the surgeon for assault and battery, and the subsequent investigation revealed many previous incidences of assault and battery, sexual harassment, and medical malfeasance that had been covered up in the past. The surgeon was relieved of duty and discharged from the army.

· · ·

PETER FISH, MD is a Major in the US Army National Guard. He served as Chief Medical Officer with the 1/101 Field Artillery Battalion in Afghanistan and as OIC Medical Affairs/Flight Surgeon with the 466 ASMC Combat Hospital in Iraq. He studied at the Army School of Health Sciences and the Army School of Aviation Medicine and is a graduate of the Physician Associate Program at Yale University School of Medicine and the Medical Doctorate Program St. George's University School of Medicine.

Part 3

IS THE PATIENT ON
THE TEAM OR NOT?

Although the three editors of this book work in health care in differing capacities—two of us as physicians, one as a writer and researcher—we share one thing in common. We have all been patients. We know all too well the fear and anxiety that we experience when we are sick and place our well-being—and indeed our lives—in the hands of strangers.

In the contemporary health care environment, patients are bombarded with supposedly reassuring messages about the care of strangers. We are told that we are now the center of care and that we will be included as members of the health care team. (Shouldn't this have always been the case?) We are now so important that surveys measure how satisfied we are and how good, or poor, our experience is with various health care institutions, providers, and workers. Most hospitals have even created an administrative post of chief of patient experience. But how does one measure the patient experience? What do patients really want? What does it mean to move from patient-centered care as a slogan to making patient-centered care a reality? How, precisely, does a patient become a part of the health care team?[1]

These are particularly vexing questions to answer since we now know that patients experience health care through very different social lenses. The overwhelming majority of patients do not have formal education in medicine or nursing or any other health profession. The average American also reads at a fifth-grade level. No matter how highly or little educated the patient is, his or her experience is determined by the subtle process of receiving and responding to social cues.[2] It doesn't take a lot of education to know whether you have been apprised of the plan for your care. You don't have to have a PhD to know whether the care process is designed around your needs or the convenience of insurers, physicians, nurses, or others in a particular health care facility. Nor does it take a lot of education to figure out whether people are talking to you or to one another about you as if you were a spectator at the drama of your illness (and thus life) while health care professionals are considered the leading actors on the stage.

Various studies—and the stories here—confirm that even the most highly educated and affluent patients are terrified of asking questions or challenging clinicians because they fear being labeled "difficult" patients.[3] Similarly, both research and narrative accounts confirm that, as Dominick L. Frosch and Susan Keim so eloquently state, even those who work in health care may find it difficult to advocate for themselves or a loved one when they or their family members are sick.[4] Indeed, ever since the publication of the book *A Taste of My Own Medicine* (popularized in the film *The Doctor*) tales of what physicians suddenly learn when they are patients has become a staple of the health care literature.[5] In these narrative accounts of the patient experience (including the one by the former *New England Journal of Medicine* editor Arnold Relman's about his care when he broke his neck) physicians describe what it feels like when they have to wait hours for a doctor—who then doesn't apologize for being late; how they are unable to protect themselves or a family member from a medical mistake; and how difficult it is for even those in the know to take responsibility for their own care or that of a loved one. Many have shared how hard it is to advocate for themselves or a loved one, even though they have great expertise and know that gaps in care may affect the clinical outcome.[6] They also describe what it means when their caregivers make an effort to listen and solicit their concerns, help ease their anxiety, and take the time to fully understand their needs and fears and provide them with information in a way they can understand.

As the stories in part 3 make clear, the only way to make sure the patient is in fact a member of the team is to take the time and energy to see things through his or her eyes by following the patient through the care experience and by inviting him or her to help design it and provide feedback about it in a meaningful way. The patient's voice always needs to be at the center of the conversation.

No, I Am Not Doing It for You

Dominick L. Frosch

In January 1988, just before I turned seventeen and while I was living in Germany, the islets of Langerhans on the surface of my pancreas stopped producing insulin. I was diagnosed with type 1 diabetes, a condition whose management in many ways exemplifies what it means to live with a chronic disease.

Successfully managing diabetes means tracking one's physiological function on a daily basis and continually adjusting and balancing insulin intake, exercise, and carbohydrate consumption. The scientific evidence is clear—if you can successfully balance all these things on a continual long-term basis, you can limit and even prevent the complications that can make type 1 diabetes so devastating.[7] But as plenty of further scientific evidence attests, engaging in the behaviors that are necessary to avoid these complications is no small task. Bodily functions you previously took for granted now require monitoring and intervention 24/7, 365 days of the year. There is no day off.

As I would later learn through my research on shared decision making and patient engagement, I was fortunate enough to have received my initial diagnosis and treatment in a German hospital that was very forward thinking. The Diabetes Control and Complications Trial (widely known as the DCCT), a clinical study that provided the strongest evidence that intensive self-management could limit and prevent complications of type 1 diabetes, would not be published until 1993, five years after my diagnosis.[8] Yet, after I was stabilized on an insulin regimen, I participated in a weeklong training program whose working assumption was that if I knew how to self-manage and keep my blood glucose levels as normal as possible, I could avoid the complications. From day one I was taught that managing my diabetes on a daily basis was not something my physician or other health care professionals would do. It was in my hands. This made sense to me. I don't live in a doctor's office, nor was I particularly interested in spending a lot of time in one.

Over thirty years ago psychologists described the concept of self-efficacy—that is, the belief that one is able to perform a particular behavior.[9] The training program I went through instilled in me the belief that I was able to do the things that were necessary to manage my diabetes and gave me the confidence to manage my condition. Higher levels of behavioral self-efficacy have been repeatedly linked to better outcomes in diabetes and other chronic diseases. And this has certainly been true in my case.

Much has been written about how to engage and motivate patients to make the behavioral changes necessary for successfully managing a chronic disease. Some of my own work as a researcher has touched on this. Wagner's chronic care model assumes that interprofessional teams coordinating care are better suited at guiding and motivating patients than single physicians.[10] But lost in all this is *how* any member of the team of health care professionals *interacts* with the patient— the most important member of the team. Over time, I've encountered, again and again, how my conception of a health care team—with me as the patient at the center—is often not shared by the health care professionals I consult with for my treatment. These people often do not communicate well with one another. Despite several decades of scholarship on interprofessional teams and attempts to advance this approach in practice, the reality is that US health care for the most part is still dominated by power hierarchies and a lack of true teamwork in which each member is clearly recognized as making an equally valuable contribution toward the goal of providing high-quality patient care. What is more troubling is that these teams also fail to communicate with me and put me at the center.

This has been highlighted in the way one of my physicians dealt with one of the most frightening risks of my disease. Diabetes remains a leading cause of preventable blindness, and as someone who loves to travel—to *see* the world—knowing this has been an important motivator encouraging me to stay on top of managing my diabetes.

Every year I schedule an appointment with an ophthalmologist to determine whether I show any evidence of diabetic retinopathy. Chronically high blood glucose leads to microaneurisms in the retina, which, left unmanaged, can leak, leading to visual impairment and, left untreated, blindness. The week before my annual ophthalmology exam is always an anxious time, as I fear that the first shoe will drop—that I will have the first signs of retinal damage—signaling the beginning of a gradual deterioration of my visual acuity.

Three years ago, I saw an ophthalmologist I hadn't seen before. After the technicians conducted the initial examinations, I sat in the room waiting for my eyes to dilate. Fifteen minutes later the physician entered the exam room, introduced herself, turned down the lights, and began her careful examination of my retinal background. For what seemed like an eternity—to me the anxious patient—she quietly conducted the exam not saying a word. Finally, she was finished, pushed back the contraption on which my chin rested and said, "Everything looks great. I don't see any trace of retinopathy." What a relief, I thought, more evidence that I must be doing the right things in managing my diabetes. But what followed next startled me as the physician said, seemingly wanting to praise me for all my effort: "You must be really good at following orders!"

For a brief moment I considered my retort. I imagined lecturing the physician on what it means to be patient centered and mentioning some papers I had written. But, instead of confrontation, I chose to just nod and smile, behaving just like many of the patients I have described in some of my research on how patients perceive interacting with physicians about medical decisions.[11] Later that night I replayed the situation in my mind and kept asking, "Do you really think I do this for *you*?" I don't check my blood glucose eight times per day to make my physician happy. I do it because it helps me make sure that I can stay on track with *my* goals, being able to travel and continue seeing the world.

The ophthalmologist probably meant well, yet her comment seemed like the perfect way to undermine my sense of achievement and self-efficacy. In her formulation, my success in staving off retinopathy was not so much my accomplishment but was instead a result of following wisely determined doctor's orders. The words she used reflect an attitude and culture that still seems all too common among many health care providers—that they are the experts and that patients need to follow orders. Other experiences, however, have shown me that physicians are not necessarily the most expert at managing my condition. Last year, when my glycohemoglobin A1c result came back at 6.7 percent, my physician e-mailed me stating that this reflected "adequate control." I, on other hand, was quite happy. For one thing, this was below the guideline target of 7.0 percent. Furthermore, it had been at or near this level for as long as I had records (in fact never reaching 7.0% or above), which, given my continued lack of retinopathy or other complications, suggested to me that this level of control is sufficient. Occasionally, in the more distant past, it has been lower, at one point coming down to 5.8 percent, almost the level you would expect to see from someone who doesn't have diabetes. But the consequences of driving my blood glucose that low went beyond helping prevent complications from diabetes.

The flip side of tight glucose management, which has been well documented in the research literature, is that it increases the risk of hypoglycemia.[12] Low blood sugar is the acute risk that a person with diabetes has to live with every day. On balance, I prefer a low blood sugar to a high one, but there are real limits and real risks. When severe hypoglycemia strikes in the middle of the night, it can lead to seizures and death. I've experienced nocturnal seizures and injured my shoulder during the last severe hypoglycemia bout I had ten years ago. I know that I don't want to take that risk anymore. Having spent more time with my primary care physician than my ophthalmologist, I decided to reply to her comment. I clarified the risks of pushing my glucose lower. I explained that for me a result of 6.7 percent was right on the sweet spot (no pun intended). My primary care physician was gracious enough to reply that she stood corrected.

How many patients would dare to push back like that? Some of my research has shown that patients often don't dare disagree with their physician's assessment because they fear it will lead to them being labeled difficult, and therefore it might compromise their care in the future.[13] Perhaps I'm a "difficult" patient. But I'm willing to live with that for the sake of my own health.

During my most recent ophthalmology exam, my twenty-fifth, which again confirmed that I must be doing something right as I still have no trace of retinopathy, the technician who began my exam made another startling remark. The process began with some questions about the past year—had I noticed any changes in my vision, did I continue to take my prescribed medicines? I answered "no" to the first question and "yes" to the second. The technician sat down in front of me, readying one of her instruments for the first part of the exam, and said, "Now we're going to see whether you are telling the truth." Why would I lie? Wasn't I there for my own sake to make sure my eyes were still in good health? It felt as though the notion that patients are to follow health care professionals' orders was rearing its ugly head again.

We've made progress in recognizing the centrality of patients in the health care team over the past twenty years. Patient engagement is an increasingly important priority for health care policy and delivery. But, at every level, we still have a long way to go in changing the attitudes of health care professionals toward patients. As the person who manages my disease every day, I want to be recognized as the most important member of the team, as the person who knows the most about what it means to live with this disease. I also want to be recognized for the fact that I'm willing and able to manage it. I don't follow orders; I don't do this for anyone but me; and I don't lie about my condition. I hope that someday my health care will be delivered by a genuine team that will have the respect and humility to understand this.

· · ·

DOMINICK L. FROSCH, PhD is a fellow in the Gordon and Betty Moore Foundation's Patient Care Program. He oversees the foundation's activities related to advancing patient and family engagement in health care. He also is an Associate Professor of Medicine at UCLA and consulting investigator at the Palo Alto Medical Foundation Research Institute. His clinical research has focused on shared decision making and patient engagement for over a decade. He has published over seventy-five peer reviewed articles and chapters and serves as deputy editor for the *Journal of General Internal Medicine*.

We're Not Listening

Michael Leonard

There's an old adage in medicine—"If all else fails, listen to the patient." I learned about this the hard way some years ago as a young anesthesiologist. I was covering a hospital obstetrical service and was called to put an epidural in for a young woman in labor; she was a short, very obese eighteen-year-old having her first child. Placing the epidural was technically difficult because of the patient's anxiety, which inhibited her ability to cooperate, and because of all her soft-tissue swelling from the pregnancy. With the hub of the five-inch epidural needle pushed against the skin of her back with some force, I was just able to reach the desired epidural space and place the catheter, which worked well for about two hours before it became dislodged. The patient's marked soft-tissue swelling and obesity also made keeping the catheter in place really difficult. The patient ultimately had three epidurals placed in the eight hours prior to her delivering a healthy baby boy. This young mother did not wish to breast-feed, so she was placed on medication to prevent lactation; otherwise she had routine postpartum care.

As we rotated one day out of every three on obstetrics, I was not on service two days later when one of my anesthesia colleagues called to ask about my care of this patient predelivery. The patient was now complaining of headaches, with visual symptoms appearing beforehand, that she described as incapacitating. The headaches seemed to last several minutes and then cease. The nurses noted the patient seemed quite normal after these episodes and began to doubt the patient's story. "Making stuff up about the patient" is a uniformly bad thing to do, but it took on a life of its own in this case. The nurses decided the patient was an "unfit mother," as she was reportedly seen trying to feed her newborn french fries. There were lots of aspersions cast: "She didn't seem to be bonding with the baby;" "She probably doesn't want to take it home;" "The headaches probably aren't real." All of this made it very hard to know what was really going on.

I told my anesthesia colleague that, though the multiple epidural placements had been difficult, I was quite sure that none of her complaints, including the possibility of a spinal headache from accidentally putting the needle in too far, was related to the anesthetic. In fact, the patient's obesity precluded putting the needle in too far, as it would just barely reach the desired space. My colleague seemed to agree.

Some hours later my anesthetic colleague called back to say, "I know you said she didn't have a spinal headache, and her symptoms didn't seem typical (the headache being worse with sitting or standing), but she has this headache. I had to do something so I gave her an epidural blood patch (injecting some of the patient's blood into the epidural space to seal the presumed leak of spinal fluid)." This was not good. The situation got even worse. My colleague continued, "It was really, really hard to find the epidural space, so I injected 30 ml of blood somewhere in her back—not really sure where." The real subtext of this conversation was: "You were there and took care of her and told me what happened, but I decided you were probably wrong so I treated a problem she probably doesn't have and did a lousy job."

The following morning I was back on the OB service and stopped in to see the patient, who still was having episodic disabling headaches preceded by this "funny light—kind of yellowish." The nurses had decided the patient had psychiatric issues and were doing their best to convince the doctors she was a head case. The doctors didn't really know what was going on, and the patient was still suffering. The least helpful physician was the consultant neurologist, who, in a seriously arrogant manner, informed me that he had decided I was wrong, the patient clearly had a spinal headache, and he instructed my colleague to treat the patient for this. He didn't have any very good answers as to why the patient's problem was unresolved. Nor did he respond to my observation that solutions built on faulty premises are generally ineffective. "Sometimes, life is not simple" was the best he could muster.

By the following morning the nurses had convinced the doctors to get a psychiatric consult to prove the patient was both a head case and an unfit mother. I came by the unit to see the patient, and while I was in the room talking with her and her husband, she had a grand mal seizure. Crazy people don't seize. People with very unhappy brains do seize. We effectively treated the seizure by helping her breathe and giving the appropriate medicines to stop it. Afterward, she was awake and talking. About this time the lightbulb in the obstetrician's head went off, and he noted the medicine he had prescribed for suppressing breast milk was reported to cause neurologic problems. When I began to read the PDR description of the bromocriptine the patient had been taking, her symptoms were a textbook description. She had been telling us with uncanny accuracy what the problem was, and we didn't listen to her.

Bromocriptine is related to ergot, and similar syndromes have been reported since the Middle Ages due to wheat contaminated with ergot. She had vasculitis, an inflammation of the blood vessels in her brain. The neurologist, not to be left out of the equation, insisted she needed an immediate angiogram of her brain. I noted that we had a clear explanation for her symptoms, that the angiogram had a 1 percent chance of causing her to stroke—squirting dye through inflamed, spasming blood vessels is best avoided, if possible—and the patient probably would be best served by stopping the medicine and watching. Predictably, she was hustled off to radiology, her angiogram showed central nervous system vasculitis, and thankfully she had no complications.

Just to insure I got to relive this all over again, when the patient sued the hospital and the drug company to avoid a somewhat crushing financial obligation, I was subpoenaed as a fact witness and deposed for five hours. Mine was the only legible handwriting in the chart.

There are two important lessons that have served me quite well since. Never ever make stuff up about patients. It's not only disrespectful but extraordinarily dangerous. The bias we allowed to be introduced into the social dynamic impaired our ability to solve the problem in an effective and timely manner. The other lesson is to always listen to patients. This young woman, who just wanted to take her baby home, very accurately and repetitively gave the information we needed. Our inability to listen to her and each other prolonged the problem and put her at great risk.

· · ·

MICHAEL LEONARD, MD is Managing Partner of Safe and Reliable Healthcare, Adjunct Professor of Medicine at Duke University, and a faculty member at the Institute for Healthcare Improvement, Cambridge, Massachusetts.

Captain, You Need to Go

Susan Keim

It was one of the hardest decisions I've had to make in my life, and, in hindsight, I believe that it was the right one. It was not, however, made easier by the circumstances. My father had a large embolic stroke two weeks earlier and, as a family, we were faced with making decisions about the end of his life. There were some complicating circumstances. My father had remarried after my mother died a few years ago, and his current spouse, Jane, had his medical power-of-attorney (POA). She was a difficult person and possessive regarding *all* matters related to my father. Although I really knew my father's wishes, I had to acquiesce to and coddle his wife, which added even more strain to the situation. I am a nurse practitioner who also worked for years in health care administration. I have some understanding regarding health care systems, but I wasn't prepared for how broken the system is and how much it affects important decisions.

After my father had emergency surgery to extract the blood clot and an intensive care unit stay that included daily CT scans, consults with cardiology and gastroenterology, and discussions with a myriad of neurologists and neurosurgeons, the conclusion was that there would be no meaningful recovery for him. Almost no one, however, was willing to be frank, and all skirted questions regarding his likely level of function. Perhaps because providers did not want to squelch any hope and also because they have seen other patients unexpectedly recover, it was difficult for them to predict my father's course. Every day a different neurologist visited my father, and because this was a teaching hospital, there was an endless stream of new faces. Even though it was hard to feel a sense of continuity, I questioned each one regarding his or her opinion of my father's prognosis. Most responses were understandably evasive since it was still relatively early in my father's course of illness. I also had to balance my questions with sensitivity to how much information Jane could handle and in deference to her stridently held position as the sole decision maker.

By this point, my father was no longer in the intensive care unit, and although it appeared that he recognized us, he was greatly compromised. He could only move his left hand and leg; and because he was aphasic, he was unable to speak to us, write, or even point to letters of the alphabet to spell out words. He could not reliably follow commands; he would give us the thumbs up sign and squeeze our hands, but that was the extent of his ability. He was incontinent of urine and stool, and he was unable to eat or swallow without risk of aspiration, so he was receiving intravenous nutritional support. Nurses streamed in and out of my father's room offering episodic care, but no one discussed potential next steps. Yet I knew we were reaching the end of the acute care phase of his illness and entering into the long-term care realm. In other words, it would soon be time to transfer out of the hospital, and I knew that couldn't happen until nutritional support could be given via a less invasive method, for example, a G-tube—a feeding tube that would be inserted in the abdomen to feed him.

At eighty-one, before the embolism, my father had been a vibrant man who loved to travel, eat in fine restaurants, traipse into New York City from northern New Jersey to see shows, take daily walks, volunteer in a hospital, play the saxophone, and tinker with his iPhone, camera, laptop, and the like. As my youngest daughter would say, "Grandpa didn't walk like a grandpa!"

To languish in bed or, at best, to be propped in a wheelchair and to lose the ability to eat independently would be devastating for most, but it would definitely not work for my father. My father truly had a love affair with food, and the thought of artificial nutrition alone would greatly reduce the quality of his life. Jane vacillated between wanting to "do everything to help him recover" and recognizing that he might never return to a level of functioning that would make him happy. I understood these conflicting emotions, and felt them too, but I knew we were running out of time to make a decision.

Finally, we were told about next steps, including the placement of a G-tube and the need to transfer my father to a skilled nursing facility (SNIF) for rehabilitation. This was explained to us in a matter-of-fact fashion as though it were an unquestionable next step. Only because I work in the health care field did I understand that we were at an important crossroads. To consent to the insertion of this tube would pave the way for his transfer. Yet, the path for the next phases of care had not been fully explained, and Jane did not understand the implications. I gently suggested that she request a family meeting with the social worker, internal medicine and neurology staff, and my husband and me. I hoped that this meeting would provide her with more information, since she clearly stated it would be her decision.

I had no idea whether she would follow through on this suggestion, so I knew I had to candidly explain the magnitude of this decision she would make. I shared with her a discussion that I had with an insightful neurology resident in the quiet hours of one evening at my father's bedside. When discussing the recent push to place a G-tube, he wisely stated that "it was easier to never put something in than it is to have to remove it later." What I had to explain to Jane (that no one in the health care team had done) was that once the G-tube is placed and my father transferred to the SNIF, my father would have to make meaningful and rapid progress in his rehabilitation or Medicare would not reimburse for his care and he would be moved to long-term care, a.k.a, a nursing home. I knew the perils of being immobilized in a nursing home, including bed sores, all types of infection, and, if my father had any cognitive awareness, likely depression. I could not imagine a more horrible way for my father to exist. This would be the antithesis of how he had lived his life. I felt, at times, that I was being harshly candid with Jane, but I knew she must understand the entire picture if she was to make a truly informed decision. She had slowly begun to involve me and my brother in decisions, I believe, because it was so overwhelming for her.

To my relief, Jane scheduled the family meeting, and, as my husband and I travelled to the hospital, we discussed the need to advocate for what we truly hoped were my father's wishes. I thought I knew what he wanted, but since he had remarried, we hadn't recently discussed these matters as Jane had made it clear she was "in charge." My father had given her POA, so he must have had faith in her. I also knew he avoided conflict, and the decision to legally give her this authority was likely his acquiescence to her forceful personality. He had written an advance directive, which Jane had not shared with us; I asked her to bring it to the meeting.

We arrived at a family lounge on the hospital unit; Jane had not brought the advance directive with her but acknowledged that she knew my father's wishes and implied that I had not incorrectly described them. My father's internist, Dr. Galloway; the chairman of the Department of Neurology, Dr. Singh (whom I had never yet seen at my father's bedside); and the social worker, Ms. Harris, came into the room. Dr. Singh authoritatively launched into the plan to have a G-tube inserted and said my father would be immediately transferred to a SNIF for rehabilitation.

"Do you believe that my father can progress in his rehabilitation? He cannot reliably follow commands," I asked him.

Dr. Singh looked annoyed and stated that my father could follow commands since he could squeeze his hand. I tried to tactfully point out that my father also "squeezes your hand when asked to follow most any other command." I asked him what he believed to be my father's (and Jane's husband's) chance for a meaningful recovery? What was his likely prognosis? What were our options if we elected to not place the G-tube?

He looked incredulous and stated that "there were no other options" and I would have to face the hospital ethics committee if we elected not to place the G-tube. I responded that, in fact, my father had an advance directive, and it was not his wish to be sustained through artificial nutrition. We would not need to face an ethics committee if we did not consent to the insertion of a G-tube. At this point, the atmosphere in the room was tense, but I felt like I was fighting for my father's life. No one else had yet spoken, but I could see Ms. Harris gently shaking her head when Dr. Singh mentioned going to the ethics committee.

Dr. Singh asked, "Why am I here at this meeting? You don't seem to want my opinion. Do I need to be here anymore?" I turned to Jane and my husband and asked them if they had any further questions for Dr. Singh. They said they didn't, and I thanked Dr. Singh and told him, "We have no further questions. You provided us your opinion

regarding his prognosis, and we no longer need you at the meeting."
He got up and walked out.

There was a collective sense of relief once Dr. Singh left the room.
Dr. Galloway concurred that my father would not wish to live in such
a compromised state, and Ms. Harris confirmed that there was no
need to confer with the ethics committee. We discussed the other care
options, which included no G-tube insertion and a transfer to short-
term acute care inpatient hospice for supportive care. Ms. Harris offered to reach the hospice admissions coordinator, and Jane agreed.

My father lived for another week and received supportive care on
the hospice unit. He never appeared to be in pain, and he slowly lost
consciousness. His family was with him when he died. I don't want
to give the impression that I always felt completely sure about our
decisions, because none of us have a crystal ball. Oddly enough, Jane
never produced the advance directive even when requested to do so
by the hospice program. I do not believe this was because she was
concealing anything but rather because she did not know how to lo-
cate it. I do believe that we acted in accord with what we knew to be
my father's wishes, and I feel like he was spared a much more difficult and protracted death.

Throughout this experience, I wrestled with not only my personal
pain but also with the anger that I felt about how unnecessarily difficult the process was, in large part, because of the lack of a cohesive
and communicative health care team. Because I understood the vaga-
ries of our health care system, I could forcibly advocate for my father.
Most families would not think they could disagree with a department chair nor could they understand the likely consequences of
care planning. Most families would not understand the importance
of the G-tube insertion decision, or the probability that short-term
rehabilitation failure would make it necessary to transfer to a nursing home. These decisions are too often made while families are
emotionally having to come to terms with the probability of there
being little chance for recovery while not yet able to acknowledge it
even as a possibility. The way in which our health care system is
structured promotes fragmented care. Physical transfers, rotating
staff, discomfort in prognosticating, lack of a "big picture" mentality,
the occasional lack of empathy, perhaps even a lack of understanding

about how financial systems influence care all converge to make difficult decisions more difficult and ill informed.

I am at peace now with the decision we made regarding my father's plan of care, but I feel no comfort in knowing that other families are victims of our health care system with its lack of teamwork. I feel badly for other patients and families who, lacking understanding of likely progression of care and knowledge of options, make decisions that result in undue hardship on all. I think about the patients who are unnecessarily languishing in nursing homes. Had their families received complete, thorough, and empathetic information from the health care team, different decisions might have been made.

· · ·

Susan Keim, CRNP is the Program Director for the Nursing and Health Care Administration and Health Leadership programs at the University of Pennsylvania School of Nursing, where she teaches a graduate course entitled "Systems Thinking in Patient Safety" and oversees the patient safety and health care quality improvement minor. She is also a practicing adult primary care nurse practitioner at a family practice in Philadelphia.

Virginia's Knee

Julia Hallisy

Few patients have looked forward to having knee-replacement surgery as much as my dental patient Virginia. Virginia is a vibrant, incredibly energetic octogenarian who is an avid ballroom dancer with her devoted husband of over fifty years. While she didn't relish the idea of surgery, she wasn't about to let her deteriorating knee joint keep her from continuing to enter ballroom dancing competitions.

I explained to Virginia that she would need antibiotic prophylaxis before her next visit in my dental office to protect her new joint from infection. When Virginia asked why she would need antibiotics, I explained in detail that bacteria from the oral cavity could enter the bloodstream during a dental cleaning and settle in her new joint and cause an infection. Virginia was surprised to learn that an infection in her new joint could ultimately necessitate the removal of the implant and lead to a delayed recovery.

Virginia understood that taking the antibiotics would lessen her odds of infection, and she promised to speak to her physician. We entered the premedication reminder in our electronic medical record and in our e-mail appointment reminder system. We had a plan.

When I next saw Virginia a few months later, she let us know that she had followed through, as she proudly held up a prescription bottle and said that she had taken one pill an hour before her appointment. I asked to see the bottle as I immediately had doubts that one pill would be a sufficient dose.

The bottle label read: "Levaquin 250 mg. Take as directed."

At first glance I assumed Virginia had simply grabbed the wrong bottle as she left her house. Virginia is allergic to penicillin, so the drug of choice for her antibiotic prophylaxis is Clindamycin.

"Virginia, are you sure that this is the medication the doctor prescribed for you to take after your knee replacement?" I asked.

"Oh, yes, I'm sure. It's the bottle from Dr. Smith—the one with the pink pills."

"Is Dr. Smith your surgeon?"

"No, he's my primary care doctor. I mentioned your comments about needing antibiotics to him and he gave me this prescription."

"How did you know how many pills to take, Virginia?" I continued my questions. "There are no specific directions on the label."

"Well, I wasn't completely sure. I didn't want to take too much, so I decided to take one."

Now I had an all-too-familiar dilemma in my practice—another provider moving forward with a medication or a dosage that was not within recommended established guidelines. I decided that I needed to stop and consult with Virginia's primary care doctor to ask about his rationale for prescribing Levaquin instead of Clindamycin. I also called my local pharmacist to ask if he was seeing orthopedic surgeons prescribing Levaquin instead of the usual antibiotic regimen recommended by the American Heart Association. As I suspected, the pharmacist was surprised at the prescription and found it as concerning as I did.

I was successful at reaching Virginia's physician, and I asked him if there was a specific reason why he prescribed Levaquin instead of Clindamycin. I was a bit taken aback at his response since I was still assuming that there had been some sort of mix-up.

"Well, the patient's allergic to penicillin, and I prefer Levaquin, anyway. That stuff kills everything. I give it to everyone," he told me.

I had to immediately switch gears as I realized that there had been no mistake, as the physician fully intended to prescribe Levaquin. I responded, "When a patient is allergic to penicillin I turn to the next appropriate antibiotic, which is Clindamycin. I'm also curious about the dose of Levaquin you are recommending since there are no specific directions on the bottle."

"Just give her the Levaquin. How many pills are in the bottle? That's probably the dose she's supposed to take," the physician responded. He was pleasant enough but clearly busy and anxious to get off the phone.

I politely extricated myself from the call and returned to speak to Virginia. I didn't want to come between my patient and the trust she had in her primary care physician, but my professional and ethical duty was to adhere to the recognized standards of care.

"Virginia, I have a bit of a predicament, and I want us to figure it out together and come to a decision we are both comfortable with. I have a specific protocol that I follow when deciding which antibiotic to prescribe for joint-replacement patients, and the one I use is recommended by organizations such as the American Heart Association and the American Academy of Orthopaedic Surgeons. Since you are allergic to penicillin, the next drug of choice for you is Clindamycin."

I saw an immediate look of recognition on her face.

"Oh, that sounds so familiar. I have had other doctors prescribe that medication because I'm allergic to penicillin," she exclaimed.

I had to admit that I breathed a little sigh of relief because it seemed that Virginia might feel comfortable accepting my recommendation. Fortunately, I wouldn't have to take a hard stand and refuse to proceed if she wanted to use an antibiotic that did not meet accepted standards of care.

"I would feel better using the one that you recommend—the one that all the groups say to use," she said.

"I would like to use Clindamycin," I responded. "And the next time you see the surgeon why don't you ask his opinion as well."

Fortunately, this went well. But what would I have done if the patient did not agree with my recommendation? I would have rescheduled her appointment and had a more involved conversation with her physician explaining that I'm not comfortable going outside the American Heart Association guidelines, and I would have asked him to consider changing his prescription. If there was still a disagreement, I would have consulted the orthopedic surgeon for his or her input. I also make a point of regularly consulting with pharmacists, as I find their detailed knowledge of medications invaluable.

Ultimately, including the patient in the final decision was both appropriate and successful. Clinicians sometimes allow their personal preferences for medications or treatment to dictate the course, when the individual needs of the patient must come first. In this situation, Virginia understood that there was a difference of opinion between her providers, listened to the rationale for my decision, weighed the evidence that was presented to her, and felt comfortable making a decision.

. . .

Julia Hallisy, DDS received her training at the University of California at San Francisco School of Dentistry in 1989 and has a full-time private practice in San Francisco, California. Her late daughter, Katherine Eileen, was diagnosed at five months of age with bilateral retinoblastoma, and dealing with the life-threatening diagnosis, the many recurrences of cancer, and the subsequent treatments for the malignant and aggressive tumors marked the beginning of a twenty-year involvement in improving our health care system. She is the founder of the Empowered Patient Coalition nonprofit organization, which works to inform, empower, and engage patients and families.

Dangerous Assumptions

Catherine Skowronsky

Recently, my big brother was hospitalized with newly diagnosed liver cirrhosis. As the "nurse in the family," I was proactive about being involved in his care. Actually, I was downright assertive about it. What good is thirteen years of health care experience if it can't be used to help my own family?

Recognizing the importance of self-care to manage chronic illness, I was careful to take time to educate my brother about his new medications. I took into consideration his independent (read stubborn) nature and lack of medical background. Then I brought to bear the knowledge I acquired as a nurse and patient educator. Our teaching session went like this: "This pill is called lactulose. You won't like it because it makes you poop. It takes the poison out of your blood that your liver can't remove anymore. If you stop, you will get confused and loopy. Don't stop taking it. This one is called lasix. You won't like it because it makes you pee a lot. Keep taking it or your ankles will swell up again and that fluid will build up in your lungs too. Remember how hard it was to breathe? Don't stop taking it." After each instruction, he would reply, "Okay, I won't stop."

At home he continued to rebound to his old self. Even down to his same old jokes. Two weeks later my sister called to tell me he was in the emergency room because "he wasn't acting right." A few hours and a few phone calls later, his lab reports revealed an elevated ammonia level. My sister and I together verified that he had stopped taking his lactulose. He had stopped all of his medications. Why? "I ran out," he told us matter-of-factly. "What am I supposed to do, take these the rest of my life?"

Yes, by all means! That is what he was supposed to do. Isn't that what I said? I told him liver damage was permanent. I explained how the liver removed poisons like ammonia. I told him the lactulose would help do that job. How did he not connect the dots and deduce that taking the medication was a lifelong commitment? Better yet, how did *I* miss filling that gap in his understanding for him?

This was a lightbulb moment for me. Nurses are supposed to decrease pain and suffering and also the length of hospital stay by effectively teaching patients about their medications. Here I was teaching someone I knew well, and still it wasn't enough to give him everything he needed to manage his illness.

What was even more amazing was that I was the first to attempt to do this. I guess it's just typical of being a nurse that I identified the gap and filled it without even thinking about who should have done this sooner. My brother spent a week in a facility for physical rehabilitation after discharge from the hospital. My initial teaching session with him took place when he was preparing to leave the rehab facility. The nurses in the hospital apparently assumed they did not need to teach him about his illness because the rehab staff would take care of that. After one week at the facility, he was forty-eight hours away from discharge, and I was still the first person to even discuss medications or disease management with him. No one had clearly explained—and made sure he understood—that he had a lifelong condition. Everyone assumed someone else would do it. But no one did, until I did. And even I failed to be fully helpful on that first try.

Fortunately, he had a nurse for a sister, and luckily I reflected enough to understand my own limitations in helping educate him. But what if, like many people, he had no health care professional in the family? Would anyone, in what was undoubtedly a busy emergency room, have realized that he did not understand the ramifications of his condition and made sure he understood that he would have to take his meds forever? What I realized is that we make all kinds of assumptions about what the people we care for understand and don't understand. We know something so we assume they do too. But if the patient is really going to be at the center of the health care team, we need to do better. We have to understand them rather than assuming they understand us.

· · ·

CATHERINE SKOWRONSKY, RN is a Clinical Nurse Specialist with the Cleveland Clinic Hospital in Cleveland, Ohio. She is a certified medical surgical nurse with thirteen years of nursing experience with the chronically ill. She utilizes her expertise in the APN role to improve nurse-physician communication.

Part 4
PSYCHOLOGICAL SAFETY

Although patients will never be safe until those who care for them feel free to voice a concern, prevent a mistake, or ask for help, advice, or clarification from their colleagues when needed, thousands—perhaps even millions—who work in health care report that they are nonetheless hesitant to speak up. Safety-culture data reveal that 20 percent of people caring for patients in the United States are hesitant to say anything when they see something that jeopardizes patient safety. One study showed an even higher percentage along with team members who reported seeing the same mistakes happening repeatedly with no way to surface and resolve them.[1] In some clinical units the number of those who are afraid to speak up about patient safety approaches as much as 50 percent. The AHRQ Hospital Survey on Patient Safety Culture found that 55 percent of respondents had not reported a single patient safety event in the past twelve months.[2] In one study of operating room personnel using the Safety Attitude Questionnaire, on average 43.4 percent of staff agreed with the statement "In this clinical area, it is difficult to speak up if I perceive a problem with patient care."[3]

Many who work in health care say they feel unsupported by their managers—particularly if they are lower on the totem pole and are challenging so-called superiors.[4] They report that their concerns may be dismissed and that they may even be disciplined for voicing them. They say they are disheartened by the incivility and disrespect that seems endemic in the health care workplace.[5] Indeed, one of the mantras of medicine and nursing (the two largest professions in health care) seems to be that doctors and nurses eat their young.

Studies suggest that members of both professions insist that they would leave the workforce if they could.[6] This makes it difficult for people to work together to create a plan of care, consider course changes and corrections, or suggest much-needed alterations in work organization.

Studies almost too numerous to cite also document that those who work in health care are afraid to admit to mistakes, which makes it difficult to learn from them.[7] Rather than being rewarded for reflecting on practice and directly acknowledging deficiencies or problems in work organization, those who work in health care are rewarded for workarounds or "first-order thinking" that addresses an immediate need but leaves in place the fundamental defect so others will have to deal with the same problem later. Anita Tucker and Amy Edmondson have noted that nurses spend as much as 15 percent of their time working around system defects to solve a problem in the short term even if that means shifting it to another clinician, unit, or health care facility.[8] The two primary factors affecting willingness to speak up are the experience someone had the last time he or she actually spoke up and knowing what the plan of care actually is.[9] Health care, as a culture, places great emphasis on being right and knowing the answers. No one wants to look dumb or ignorant, so knowing what is expected to happen and being invited to speak up are quite important.

As we have seen in part 2, the brain's negativity bias makes psychological safety an imperative. Few of us who have been unsupported, humiliated, or disciplined for speaking up will venture into such dangerous territory again—no matter the risk to the patient. Whether one is a team leader or member, the creation of psychological safety involves having the courage to take direct and very public action to support those who speak up.

In one way or another all the stories in this book center around the creation—or failure to create—psychological safety in the health care workplace. The stories in part 4 particularly focus on the leadership skills that are critical to making psychological safety a daily workplace reality. If there is one primary function of effective leaders it is, in our view, creating an environment where no one is hesitant to voice a concern about a patient or situation. This means leaders must set a positive, active, nonpunitive tone, share the plan, and invite team members into the conversation so that they too can share their concerns and ideas. It is reinforced when those leaders publicly stand up for staff who challenge those higher up the ladder. In other words, the job of the leader, as Michael Leonard and David L. Feldman explain, is to make it crystal clear to everyone in a unit or institution that any and every legitimate attempt to protect patients and follow policy will be supported no matter whose feathers get ruffled and how much such people complain.

Remember to Say "Please"

Martyn Diaper

My first job after graduating from medical school was as a surgical house officer in Truro, Cornwall. I had spent six years training in London and had no real career goals. I was unsure what I wanted to do and so thought I would bide my time in the west of England. I decided to get as far away from London as possible, and Cornwall was the ideal place. Situated on the far southwestern peninsula of England it offers beaches and surfing in the summertime and howling gales in the wintertime. Because it was remote from the hustle and bustle of the large population centers it was often difficult to attract medical staff to the area. I thus found myself working with some doctors who seemed like fairly colorful characters—especially to this newly qualified doctor from the city.

One such character was John. He arrived one rainy autumn day, announced by the rumble of the engine in his beat-up VW camper van. He was a well-traveled man in his early thirties, who lived, with his wife, out of the van in the parking lot throughout his two-week stay as locum surgical registrar (a fully trained surgeon filling in for someone on vacation or absent for some other reason). John was, what might be termed, a hippy. No one seemed to have told him this was the 1980s, not the 1960s. He sported a long blond ponytail and cheesecloth shirt. He wore open-toed sandals and topped it all off with the obligatory white coat. Since I had followed a very traditional English medical school career path, I initially assumed John had little to teach me. What I discovered was that, in spite of his eccentric attire, he was a man with experience beyond his years and that gentle inquiry could prize out stories of his working his way through hospitals in Africa, India, and the Far East. He was as happy delivering babies as removing an appendix or treating diabetes. He was a real Jack-of-all-trades and master of quite a few.

Late one night, I learned a lesson from John that stays with me until this day. We were looking after a very sick old man with gastrointestinal bleeding, and I was busying myself with my role of taking blood, arranging X-rays, and coordinating with the operating theater. I felt very important and on current reflection recognize that I was beginning to enjoy that sense of self-importance.

As John and I sat at the nursing station on the ward talking about the management plan for the patient, I was writing the request form for the cross matching to determine blood compatibility for the transfusion.

I just filled it in and scribbled my name on the form. To me, that was that. Not for John.

"Always write 'please' on the form," he said.

"I beg your pardon?" I replied.

"When you request any investigation, always write 'please' on the form. We often remember to say 'please' and 'thank you' to people we work with face to face, but we don't always remember to say 'thank you' to colleagues who work equally hard but whom we never see. First, if the poor lab technician has got out of bed to cross match some blood, he deserves your thanks and will feel a whole lot better about his disturbed night if he feels you are grateful. Second, if you show people that you are kind and considerate, they will be kind and considerate to you in the future. When you need their help, they will be more likely to help you. Just by using that word, 'please,' you can connect with people you never meet."

I did what he suggested. I wrote "please."

And I have been doing so ever since. To this day, I write 'please' on my request forms. It has become natural to write "chest X-ray, please," "renal ultrasound, please," or "cross match 4 units, please."

I never met John again, but his wisdom has stayed with me. I feel sure that connecting on a human level with other health care workers in the care pathway, just by saying "please," has made health care workers I communicate with feel valued. To do this routinely communicates the fact that we are caring professionals, and I hope patients receive better care because of this.

Over the years, colleagues in support services have commented that they are aware that I am respectful of their time and understand the difficult and demanding conditions under which they work. They seem to feel that the "please" they see on requests is a recognition that their work is as valuable as mine and that we are all working to get the patient better.

So my question is: Why aren't we all taught to put "please" on our requests (orders) in medical school? And how about "thank you?"

· · ·

MARTYN DIAPER, MD is a family doctor in Winchester, England. He is Clinical Lead for Safer Care for the National Health Service (NHS) Improving Quality Delivery Team, Chairman of NHS England's Patient Safety Expert Group for Primary Care, and Clinical Director for Integrated Community Services in South East Hampshire.

Getting Help When You Need It

Michael Leonard

It is hard to imagine that anyone caring for a sick, vulnerable hospitalized patient would worry that if he or she asked a "member" of his or her "team" for help that help would not be forthcoming. When I was the national physician leader for patient safety in a large integrated health system of thirty-six hospitals, I learned that this was indeed a major concern when we started doing perinatal safety training across the system. Our team of nurses, physicians, midwives, and others asked the nurses and midwives: "When you ask a physician to come to the bedside to see a patient you're concerned about, can they find a way to say no?"

Surprisingly, in hospitals where the obstetricians were physically in house, the answer was "yes."

This was a surprise because we'd invested lots of time in teaching teamwork and effective communication in our system. Yet, we nonetheless discovered that, at times, there was a lack of social agreement regarding how clinicians would respond and support one another.

The roots of this behavior are deeply embedded within the culture of medicine. Historically, we have trained doctors and nurses to be individual experts. The expectation has been that if you know what you're doing, are paying attention and trying hard, you can deliver perfect care without making mistakes. Given the premise that skilled clinicians always know the answers and can fix clinical problems, it makes it very hard for someone at the bedside to raise his or her hand and ask for help. It can be perceived as a sign of weakness or lack of competence. No one wants to look stupid, so leadership has to make it safe for people to ask for help.

The fact that some physicians had begun to engage in high-risk, self-serving behaviors was also indicative of a culture that lacked effective leadership. High-performance cultures are very clear about defining behavioral expectations and ensuring they apply to everyone. They are also quite clear about reinforcing psychological safety—the expectation is that everyone feels safe to ask for help and that they know they will receive it in a respectful way.

Thankfully, strong senior clinical leadership within the various hospitals was available to address the problem. So we went to the senior physicians at the hospital level or in obstetric departments and explained the behavioral expectations we needed if we were really going to achieve better teamwork and safer care. As the perinatal safety team, we could easily and clearly set the expectation, but without visible leadership support, we were unlikely to eliminate some long-standing tribal behaviors—where the needs of a few supersede the needs of the many.

At one of our meetings, for example, our ally was the physician-in-chief of the hospital. He made it very clear that if a nurse or midwife asked for help, physicians had better be at the bedside within minutes and needed to show up with a good attitude, that is, "How can I help you?" This was important in two respects: it conveyed the message that help was always available to assess and help solve a problem and that showing up with a bad attitude was unsafe and would destroy any sense of teamwork.

This practice became a standard part of the perinatal work in three dozen hospitals. The perinatal units embraced multidisciplinary briefings at the start of the shift so that the team knew the plan of care for each patient. Clinical leaders consistently reinforced that asking for help was welcome. Moreover, knowing the plan of care increased predictability for the nurses at the bedside who could now better understand when things with the patient were going in the right or wrong direction. Leaders continually reinforced that nurses should speak up if they had a concern. They also said that they wanted to know of any occasion in which there was a suboptimal response.

On the few occasions when this happened, senior clinical leaders dealt with them quickly and openly. In some cases, the physicians were told to go and apologize to the nurse. That sent a pretty clear message. The upside of this agreement around collaborative work was that people worked better as a team, had fewer surprises and unneeded calls, and found that it made their work easier and safer. In addition to the briefings, there was a commitment to a standardized approach to teamwork and communication using SBAR (Situation-Background-Assessment-Recommendation); quick, routine debriefings; a standardized method of interpreting and describing electronic fetal heart monitoring; and standard processes for the induction of labor, managing shoulder dystocia, and vacuum extractions. All these interventions had value, but without the commitment that it was always safe to ask for help and expect to receive it, we were building a house on an unstable foundation. What if you woke up at night in your house and smelled smoke, called 911, and the firefighters decided whether or not they wanted to leave the station?

Because of this experience, I learned not to take anything for granted about how clinical teams work together. I have since left that job and now work in hospitals as a safety expert. Working in many different hospitals, I have learned to be explicit in describing and implementing the specific behaviors that enhance teamwork. My mantra has become: Take nothing for granted. If we're going to be effective in changing behavior we have to give people explicit advice. I have learned to clearly define the behaviors that create value (effective leadership, team behaviors, comfort in speaking up, always knowing the plan) and the behaviors that create unacceptable risk (poor teamwork, not knowing the plan of care, being unresponsive or disrespectful). Safe care is all about building positive relationships among members of the care team.

Routinely, I will ask nurses whether they can always get help to the bedside and about the attitude of the people who show up. This is critical to the success of Rapid Response Teams (RRT), because it can dramatically affect the threshold to call for help. No one caring for patients wants to look dumb or incompetent, so there is an inherent threshold to seek help. The most effective hospitals have members of the RRT who don't just wait for a call but who actually round on the floors, creating relationships, seeking out nurses and taking a few minutes to talk with them about their sickest patients. Not only does this active surveillance find problems earlier but also it teaches nurses that a supportive colleague will show up to help them.

Safe care is all about trust and relationships. A negative interaction or someone saying, "Why did you bother me for this crap?" will have lasting implications because the nurses will have to be desperate before they will invite that experience in the future. Intervening early allows problems to be fixed while they are small rather than big, which is why the cultural dynamic of building relationships and making it safe to ask for help is essential. I always ask nurses whether there are physicians or other nurses they are hesitant to approach or difficult to deal with. Generally there are a few people whose names pop up pretty quickly. During training we define why this is dangerous for everyone and have leadership commit to immediately resolving the issue. Safety cannot be personality dependent—that is, possible with come colleagues but not others.

Thankfully, several hospitals have adopted the following standard: when help is requested at the bedside, a positive response is mandatory. In one new hospital the chief medical officer gathered all the clinical staff the evening before opening the new building. He stood in front of four hundred people and said, "All you physicians need to know that if you are asked to come to the bedside and see a patient, and you find a way to say no—two things will happen: one, I will be at the bedside within twenty minutes to help, and two, you will be talking to me by the following morning at the latest." This was a great way to define their culture and sent an important message that patients come first and that failure to help when a patient might be in trouble was not acceptable under any circumstance. Our people and our patients should know we are always there to help in any way.

· · ·

MICHAEL LEONARD, MD is Managing Partner of Safe and Reliable Healthcare, an Adjunct Professor of Medicine at Duke University, and a faculty member at the Institute for Healthcare Improvement, Cambridge, Massachusetts.

Liberating the Positive Deviants

Michael Gardam

Health care workers are confronted with a variety of challenges every day: some are relatively simple, such as taking a patient's blood pressure, while others can be highly complex, such ensuring patients know what medications to take when they are discharged home. In the latter example, patients may have leftover medication from other prescriptions, be taking medication given by other providers, use more than one pharmacy, have side effects, have difficulties understanding instructions in English, and so on. One can perhaps intuitively understand that the approach used to create the stepwise recipe to ensure that blood pressures are measured correctly likely cannot be simply applied to this more complex problem: there are many more variables involved, several of which may be unknown or unpredictable. The knowledge gained from the burgeoning field of health care complexity science suggests that while health care workers may want to simplify complex problems through using checklists and other tools in attempts to make them more manageable, they are often unsuccessful. Tackling complex problems requires very different approaches.

Positive Deviance is one such approach that has been used in a variety of community and institutional settings to help solve seemingly impossible complex problems. Central to this approach is the concept that within any given population, there are individuals who have developed strategies or behaviors that allow them to achieve results superior to their peers despite having access to the same resources. These "outliers" may not know that they are doing anything special and may often go unnoticed or may be suppressed by the prevalent culture that doesn't encourage local innovation or variation.

The dominant health care culture tends to be fairly hierarchical and "top down," meaning that practices and practice changes are rolled out from leadership down to frontline workers. While this approach may well work for simpler challenges, top-down strategies may ultimately fail for solving complex problems that are deeply rooted in behavior, because those asked to implement the prescribed changes may feel that they are out of touch with what they are facing on the front line. The experience with Positive Deviance and other approaches that deeply engage the groups one wants to change is that having those who are "touching the problem" implement their own solutions may ultimately result in profound, sustained improvement. This does not mean that top-down strategies can never work in health care; rather, improvement strategies need to be highly sensitive to local conditions and may involve a variety of top-down and bottom-up approaches occurring at the same time.

The Infection Prevention and Control (IPAC) program at our hospital network has used Positive Deviance for several years as part of a larger frontline health care worker empowerment approach to foster ownership of patient safety issues. Being quite counter to the traditional top-down approach learned during my medical training, it took many months for me to understand how this approach could be used to help our team in learning how to approach challenges differently, to understand the organic nature of the spread of behaviors and actions, and finally to begin to see large improvements roughly three years after we began.

One area of particular concern for our IPAC program is hospital "superbugs." These are organisms that patients typically acquire during their hospitalization that are resistant to antibiotics and may go on to cause serious infections that can be fatal. *Clostridium difficile* is a notorious superbug that has emerged over the past decade as a new, highly virulent strain and has spread around the world. *C. difficile* bacteria are first ingested. They gain entry to the mouth through contaminated hands or food and then settle in the colon where they lie dormant but ready to cause illness. Patients get sick when the bacteria begin to produce toxins that damage the lining of the intestine, which leads to pain and diarrhea in milder cases and, in severe cases, to extreme damage to the colon, septic shock, or death. *C. difficile* bacteria preys on the elderly and those with multiple other medical problems; in other words, the same population one will often find in hospitals. It is not an exaggeration to say that this organism results in the painful premature deaths of thousands of people in North America each year.

In many ways, *C. difficile* is a perfect hospital pathogen: patients' symptoms cause it to spread to others; it can live in the environment potentially for years; the illness it causes is encouraged by the gross overuse of antibiotics and drugs that block the production of stomach acid; it can readily be passed from patient to patient via health care workers' hands; and regular hospital disinfectants can't kill it. Given this perfect storm, it is not surprising that there is no one simple solution that can solve the problem. One can imagine working to get health care workers to wash their hands more often between patients yet still see the same rate of illness because the organism can still reach patients because they contaminate surfaces that they touch.

Like most North American hospitals, we have struggled to control the spread of *C. difficile*. Multiple strategies had been tried including using powerful disinfectants that can kill *C. difficile* spores but unfortunately also damage equipment. We've also worked to improve health care worker hand washing, a well-known problem that requires a surprisingly large amount of sustained work to improve. Despite these considerable efforts, *C. difficile* rates on our medicine floors at Toronto General Hospital climbed for five straight quarters, culminating in an outbreak in 2011. While we were able to contain and stop the outbreak by using aggressive temporary measures, including closing the floors to new admissions, we had reached a point where we were running out of strategies and our top-down approaches were not significantly reaching frontline workers. Central to our challenge was the fact that compliance with any one practice such as hand washing was less than ideal, and yet we knew that multiple practices had to improve if the medicine wards were going to turn the problem around. Simply put, the IPAC program knew what needed to be done, but it was the staff who needed to change their practices, many of which were deeply rooted behaviors.

In the spring of 2011 one of the internists working on the general medicine floor that had recently experienced the outbreak had a brief conversation with me about *C. difficile*. She had been deeply affected by her elderly patients becoming ill and had recently learned from the medical literature that hospital superbugs can readily live on health care workers' clothes. She wondered if her wearing surgical scrubs while providing clinical care was a good way of preventing the spread of *C. difficile* spores between patients.

As we chatted outside of the elevator, I realized how my approach to controlling infections in hospitals had changed over the past few years. Had she asked me this question three years earlier, I would have said that while there is evidence that clothing can be contaminated with a variety of hospital pathogens, there is no proof that wearing scrubs in and of itself improves patient infection rates or outcomes. Basically, whatever clothes you are wearing can become contaminated whether they are street clothes or scrubs. To be blunt, I would have told her that she was probably wasting her time.

Fortunately for our patients, I had spent several years training myself to think and approach problems differently by the time she asked me this question. The new me recognized that here was a frontline physician who wanted to start tackling a problem that desperately needed to be addressed. While there was no scientific evidence to say *C. difficile* rates would decrease, I understood that no one could predict what might happen if she started to visibly act differently. I also knew that no harm could come from her putting her idea into action. Finally, I was struck by the sobering thought that I had likely shut down many such ideas over the first ten years of my career.

I told her it was a great idea and that she had my full support to start right away. She began wearing scrubs and was immediately questioned by nurses, students, and medical and other staff as to why she had changed her clothing. On a ward full of health care workers wearing street clothes, she stood out like a sore thumb. When she responded that she was doing this to decrease *C. difficile*, it started a conversation about the seriousness of health care–associated infections and raised awareness about all the ways *C. difficile* was likely being transmitted. Instead of hearing these messages from outsiders from IPAC during an education session, staff were having natural peer-to-peer conversations. Some physicians questioned the scientific evidence behind the doctor's actions; however she felt confident that because I supported her it was the right action to take.

Over the next few months, a series of interconnected events took place that all stemmed from her decision to act differently. Having been convinced that she might be on to something, the other physicians decided to wear scrubs: soon the different medicine teams had scrubs embroidered with their team number. Residents and medical students were encouraged to join in and wear scrubs that the physicians would pay for. Friendly competition sprung up over which team could achieve the highest hand-hygiene compliance rate. I knew something remarkable was underway when I heard through the grapevine that physicians were now teaching their students about hand hygiene during their morning rounds. Independent auditors began telling me that at long last, all professions on the medicine floors were washing their hands more. Over the space of several months, the hand washing rates on the medicine floors climbed out of the basement and entered the top third of all of our programs.

The social change did not, however, stop there: the internists and other nonmedical staff decided to take a written pledge to clean their hands. Buttons started sprouting up on the unit saying, "I took a pledge." Medical students from the University of Toronto were invited to develop an internal medicine–specific hand-hygiene campaign. Although IPAC gave advice on the campaign, it was conceived, created, and led by the internal medicine program. Finally, one of the general internists, who was also an accomplished amateur filmmaker, made a simple hand-hygiene video that has subsequently been downloaded tens of thousands of times off YouTube and Vimeo.

Within a few months of the start of this cascade of frontline-led quality improvement, rates of health care–associated infections plummeted. Rates of *C. difficile* dropped over 90 percent from their all-time high. Floors that once were plagued with repeated outbreaks now rarely had even single cases of infection each month. A year later hand-hygiene rates had climbed to meet the hospital's quality improvement target, and infections are now rare. It is impossible to say which of the above interventions brought about such dramatic improvements in infection rates. Complexity science would suggest that the interventions themselves were less important than the fact that those immersed in the problem began to step outside the norm and act differently. Thus, the lesson is less that wearing scrubs will decrease infection rates than that genuine ownership and engagement of those touching the problem and allowing change to unfold can bring about remarkable improvements.

As these changes were underway, and more and more social proof was gathering that the medicine floors were doing something special, it was suggested that perhaps all medical teams in other hospitals should be required to wear scrubs. I've resisted making this recommendation because my ordering teams to change their behavior is a step backward to our old way of doing things. Wearing scrubs worked on those floors because the idea originated there: my telling other people what to do is not likely to motivate them to own improvement processes. Rather, I suggested we share the success story with other areas of the hospital and allow them to decide whether wearing scrubs works for them. Even if they choose not to adopt the strategy, they will learn of the success, and this will encourage them to try their own ideas.

The role of IPAC in this process was to step back and let it unfold. In a world of evidence-based medicine, most IPAC programs would stop such innovation before it started simply because there was little evidence to support it. Fortunately, I recognized the internist as a "positive deviant" and encouraged her to act on her idea. Complexity science recognizes that there is rarely a linear association between cause and effect. The scrubs were likely not what was important: what was really important was the visible leadership from a physician who wanted to make a difference.

· · ·

MICHAEL GARDAM, MD is an Infectious Diseases specialist and Medical Director of Infection Prevention and Control at the University Health Network in Toronto. He is a Canadian pioneer in the use of the complexity science–based behavioral change approach Front-Line Ownership to address difficult-to-solve safety problems. He has worked with health care organizations across Canada and internationally to improve patient safety.

I Should Have Said Something

Suzanne Gordon

I recently performed the play I wrote with Lisa Hayes, *Bedside Manners*, at an East Coast teaching hospital. The play includes many scenes in which physicians and nurses—and others who work in health care—fail to communicate in even the most basic way. During the discussion period that followed the play, the hospital's CEO raised his hand. "In your play," he said, "a lot of nurses are trying to raise critical issues and prevent mistakes and are blown off by physicians. That's not our main problem in this hospital. In this hospital our main problem is that nurses are too deferential and acquiescent. They see things that are about to happen that could lead to a mistake and don't say anything. What can be done about that?"

I wanted to respond with a whole lot of questions: "Why are nurses hesitant to raise their concerns? Could it be that they feel that you—as head of the hospital—have not made it clear you will support them? Have you told the nursing staff, in no uncertain terms, that any physician who chews them out will hear from you—immediately? You're the CEO. You are in charge. You had an opportunity to express your support for the nurses—and other nonphysician staff—here at this performance. Yet, you didn't turn around and ask everyone why nurses feel it is such a risk to speak up. You didn't ask nurses what they encounter when they do speak up. You didn't ask your fellow physicians why they don't encourage nurses to speak up and thank nurses when they do. And, most important, you didn't say to the group, that you want nurses and everyone in the hospital to know that when they do speak up that you—the CEO of the institution—will support them. Even if it's a wrong call, if it was made because of a concern for patient safety, you will back them up and thank them." I didn't say any of that.

Instead, I agreed that this was a problem and that it needed to be addressed and that it had to do with socialization and medical culture.

Later, in the hallway, I chatted with the CEO. He continued expressing his concerns about nurses' deference—which he had somehow constructed as a nursing problem not a problem of his leadership or that of others in top and mid-level management. Then, without connecting the issue with the one we had just discussed, he explained that some physicians were great team players and communicators. But there were others who were difficult if not downright abusive. "We are struggling. We don't really know what to do about them," was what he concluded.

And so, again, I thought but didn't say, "Well, no wonder nurses are afraid. If you don't know what to do, if you have the power and leverage and don't use it, then it's not their problem—a nursing problem—it's a failure of leadership. It's your problem."

I had nothing to lose by saying any of this—particularly if I said it in a more diplomatic way than I was thinking it. The performance was over. I would have no further contact with this institution. I would be paid for my time no matter what I said to the CEO. Yet, I didn't feel safe enough to challenge his assumptions, analysis, or interpretation of the problem. I was silencing myself. I regret that I did not have the courage to speak up. Had I done so, it might have actually helped the nurses in his institution, since modeling assertive behavior can be helpful even if you aren't connected to a particular facility. It would also have been interesting to see how the CEO responded to my comments.

I hope to learn a lesson in courage because of this encounter. Next time, in a situation in which I am a visitor in an institution asked to present about patient safety and get a question like this, I hope I have the guts and wisdom to politely say what I think. I hope to do it. But I know it will be hard. I rehearse in the shower and on walks. I just hope I get another opportunity to practice what I preach.

. . .

SUZANNE GORDON is an award-winning journalist and author who writes about health care delivery and health care systems and patient safety.

Thank You for Your Vigilance

David L. Feldman

It happened four years ago when I was in charge of perioperative services at a major medical center in New York City. My role was to manage over two hundred full-time staff and in particular to help improve the working relationships they had with the physician staffs of anesthesiologists and surgeons who were under the direction of the departmental chairmen. In that capacity, I received many phone calls, complaining, praising, and raising critical issues. So it was no surprise that I was immediately contacted about a problem that occurred between a physician and nurse in the operating room.

The patient was a seventy-six-year-old man with significant dementia who was transferred from another hospital with an acute abdominal problem. On the evening of transfer, the patient had an X-ray to confirm a diagnosis that would require a surgical procedure. A general surgeon saw the patient briefly. He viewed the radiology results and confirmed the need for an operation, which he would perform the next day. The patient's guardian consented to the procedure but was not able to be present the next day when the patient was brought to the OR, as he lived quite far from the hospital and had to attend to other family obligations.

On the morning of surgery the patient was brought to the holding area, a small room outside of the ORs where nursing and anesthesiology staff interview the patient and confirm that all paperwork has been properly completed. The circulating nurse assigned to the OR where the patient was to have surgery came to the holding area to see the patient and perform her part of the Universal Protocol. The UP is a Joint Commission requirement that includes an independent verification of the patient and procedure by each member of the surgical team (surgeon, anesthesiologist, nurse), marking of the operative site (when applicable), and a time-out immediately prior to the start of the operation.

The circulating nurse was a quiet and thoughtful woman. She had worked at the hospital for several years and was known to be sensitive and caring about patients. She did not like confrontations and had been brought to tears on several occasions when colleagues— either nurse or physician—reprimanded her for not following a policy or not being quick enough to act on a request.

The surgeon was the total opposite. He had a reputation for being loud and obnoxious; he considered himself an expert in his field and was not afraid to let people know it. The resident and nursing staff on the floors did not like working with him because he used abusive language with them. After one particularly bad occasion a couple of years earlier, he was required to attend a few sessions on sensitivity training at a large multidisciplinary conference.

When the nurse went to identify the patient, she needed to check the armband to make sure the name on the armband matched the name on the OR schedule. This was important because the patient was neither able to speak nor identify himself and, in particular, because his guardian was not able to be in the hospital for the procedure. Unfortunately, the armband did not match the patient listed on the OR schedule, and so the nurse was concerned that this was not the correct patient. By this time, the surgeon had entered the holding area and proceeded to perform his independent verification. Since he had seen the patient the previous evening, he was absolutely convinced that this was the correct patient. However, his certainty alone was not sufficient because the UP mandates an acceptable means of identification with two patient identifiers such as name, birth date, or the like.

Despite the surgeon's insistence that the patient was the correct one, the nurse prevented the patient from entering the OR until she could get clarification. She immediately contacted the nurse manager and hospital risk management. Within twenty minutes the staff concluded that another nurse had put the wrong patient armband on the patient the night before and that the patient was, in fact, the correct one to have the surgery. The patient was then brought into the OR and underwent a successful procedure.

When the nurse manager first contacted me about the situation I thought about what my response, if any, should be. At the time, most of the OR staff, including the physicians, knew that we were trying to create an environment more conducive to good teamwork. As is typically the case, some staff, both nurses and physicians, really believed in this approach. Others, as they put it, just wanted to be left alone to continue doing things the way they always did them. I thought that the surgeon probably understood that the nurse needed to follow the UP and that this was not an emergent operation and could be delayed until the problem was straightened out. He was, I believed, more cynical than combative. Nonetheless, in typical fashion, he couldn't contain his frustration and expressed his disgruntlement about these kinds of OR hiccups with anyone who would listen. The nursing staff thus considered him to be disruptive, disrespectful, and difficult to work with. These feelings are not a foundation for good OR teamwork. Silence was, for me, not an option.

My mandate was to enhance teamwork and, thus, patient safety. I knew that this was an excellent opportunity to reinforce a message we had been trying to send—that staff should speak up whenever they thought patient safety was at stake. This was especially important when they were facing someone who did not agree with their interpretation of the facts and who might be perceived as potentially threatening. I knew that this incident, if not dealt with proactively, could lead to future perfect storms in which the interpersonal problems among providers could have a profoundly negative influence on the outcome of the care of critically ill patients.

I had also known this nurse for a long time and knew she could use encouragement for doing something she was clearly not comfortable doing. Since I knew other nurses would hear about it, I also wanted them to feel that I supported this kind of action, even in the face of a physician who had a reputation for dismissing the suggestions of others.

So, after the day ended, I personally contacted the nurse and thanked her for being willing to "stop the line." I also wrote her a letter and made sure that her supervisor knew that she had contributed to making the OR a safer place for patients. Because the surgeon involved had not exhibited inappropriate behavior in this case, I didn't think it was necessary to reprimand him. However, he couldn't help but notice that the concerns of the nurse were given equal weight to his own. Not only had she stopped the line but also we applauded her for doing it. I know that he got the message because he started to behave differently. In this instance, as in so many others, my goal was not to embarrass anyone or to assign blame but rather to promote a culture of safety—something that often needs to be done one patient, one nurse, and one doctor at a time.

. . .

DAVID L. FELDMAN, MD, MBA, CPE, FACS is Senior VP and Chief Medical Officer at Hospitals Insurance Company, which provides professional liability for hospitals, physicians, and health care professionals throughout New York State.

Part 5

TEACHING WHAT
WE PREACH

$\mathbf{A}$s noted in the introduction, expert coaching is one of
the critical components of a real team. To turn a group of actors into
an ensemble, to unite disparate athletes into an effective sports team,
to weld the staff on a hospital unit into a team that exists in more than
name only involves not only a director, team owner, quarterback, or
world-renowned surgeon but also constant coaching. Whether provided by formal leaders or team members, constructively offering
and graciously receiving coaching interventions at the "appropriate"
time is a characteristic of effective teams. As Hackman and Wageman
put it, coaching is "direct interaction with a team intended to help
members make coordinated and task-appropriate use of their collective resources in accomplishing the team's work."[1] It is the essence of
making the individual resource a collective one. Thus, "coaching interventions are made at times when the team is ready for them and
able to deal with them—that is, at the beginning for effort-related
(motivational) interventions, near the midpoint for strategy-related
(consultative) interventions, and at the end of a task cycle for (educational) interventions that address knowledge and skill."[2] Coaching, in
other words, is not a one-time activity. It is a constant one.[3]

Teaching and coaching can occur in a formal manner or they can
be delivered through informal lessons when a behavior is noted, a
request made, or an interaction observed. Whatever their nature,
without teaching and coaching, no organizational intervention to
encourage teamwork will succeed. We have all watched numerous
hospitals and other health care facilities hire expensive consultants
or send their staff to programs like TeamSTEPPS and then neglect to

continue to teach and coach staff in the processes and protocols promoted by the consultant or chosen program. TeamSTEPPS specifically includes a section on coaching in its training. One of the jobs of institutional and unit-level leadership is, therefore, to make sure that coaching and teaching occur over the long term so that suggested processes become daily practice.

In these stories, coaches and teachers include both the usual and unusual suspects. Some coaching is delivered as part of a formal effort to design a "best practice" that is created by the team, for the team, and then evaluated and reported on in a published report in a peer reviewed journal. Others are based on what Michael Gardam calls "practice-based evidence" and depend on the willingness of those who are both team leaders and members to be mindful of their own responses and flexible when suggestions are made.

All the stories here reflect on the fact that health care is a complex endeavor, which means that coordination and reliable processes are essential. As we explained in part 4, health care has traditionally relied on a great deal of first-order problem solving—that is, the nurse doesn't have linen for the bed but knows where to scrounge some from another unit.[4] She is rewarded for solving the problem, but no one considers that she has just exported the problem to other nurses on another floor who cannot find bed linens when they need them.

First of all, this common problem reflects the lack of consistent mental infrastructure common to all who work in health care. It also characterizes a culture that has relied on smart people to consistently solve recurrent, avoidable problems without the mobilization of system thinking. Higher-order problem solving requires a learning system so that defects and problems are addressed and fixed and the learning is shared. This means there has to be a lot of teaching and coaching. Organizational learning provides a foundation to continually improve care and allows caregivers to feel that their input is valued and acted on.[5] In these stories, organizational learning takes place informally when a pharmacist questions a resident's order, when a nurse coaches another nurse about her approach to a physician, and when another nurse teaches a resident while both are engaged in routine patient care duties. At a more formal level, coaching and teaching occur when an entire department studies and learns from adverse events (and then takes their knowledge system-wide via a journal article) and when an entire health system begins to change practice in all its settings. Teaching and coaching also occur when practitioners reflect on their own actions, which includes the willingness to teach or coach a patient or a high-level hospital executive.

Some of the stories in part 5 may provoke a common reaction: Isn't all of this just common sense? Do we really need programs to investigate or disseminate information about something no one should have overlooked or done in the first place? How could so many people ignore things that are so self-evident? Don't people share their solutions and stories in the course of their work? The answer is that smart people do stupid things all the time and that cross monitoring and learning from even the most trivial-seeming events and activities can produce significant, even life saving, results. There is a reason that many eyes and the brains connected to them are better than one.

What the stories in this part also point to is that uncommon suspects (more on this in part 8) such as a hospital security officer, a community pharmacist, or an irate patient often have a lot to teach us. If teamwork is to be a reality we have to think outside of the conventional box when we think about teams. In an era when there is a lot of focus on interprofessional teamwork, we need to remember what Kathleen Burke reminds us, that intraprofessional teams are as important as interprofessional ones and, as Kelly Hancock and James Merlino argue, that providing safe and satisfying patient care depends not only on elite professionals but also everyone from the housekeeper to the person delivering the patient's meal tray. These people actually see a lot and know a whole lot more than they are given credit for. Perhaps the most important unusual suspect from whom we can learn is: the patient.

Learning When the Team Fails

Harry C. Sax

"The wrong-side surgeries at Rhode Island Hospital are a wake up to all of us. We are as vulnerable as anyone, despite the work we've done with checklists and crew resource management. Be alert and take advantage of each other's expertise."

I wrote this note in my role as chief of surgery at the Miriam Hospital (TMH) in Providence six weeks before we had a wrong-side surgery.

It shouldn't have happened. I had prided myself that we were engaging all members of the staff at Miriam Hospital in the concepts of optimal team functioning, communication, and the use of a surgical checklist before any invasive procedure. We were part of the same medical enterprise, Lifespan, as Rhode Island Hospital (RIH) and believed we had been proactive in our approach to patient safety. RIH had experienced a series of wrong-side procedures, and we were all trying to figure out what we could do to prevent the next one. TMH was a smaller hospital and thus able to serve as a test bed for initiatives such as using checklists and adopting institution-wide crew resource management training. The checklists were designed by a team that included staff from nursing, anesthesia, surgery, radiology, and quality improvement. Their use was monitored, and the scrub tech would not hand up the knife until the list was complete, including the surgical pause. There was an institutional sense of pride that we had minimized our chances of error.

In a cruel twist of fate, I was invited away to the University of Indiana as visiting professor to lecture on our success with operating room checklists and team training. As I was giving my talk, back in Rhode Island one of our orthopedic surgeons did something we believed we had guarded against: he inserted an arthroscope and performed a procedure on the wrong knee of a patient. The error wasn't discovered until the patient awoke in the recovery room and screamed,

"My God, they operated on the wrong knee!" The newspapers were calling within hours, and my CEO was beside herself with shock and disbelief.

We immediately shifted into mitigation mode. We spoke to the patient and the patient's spouse as well as the operative team. Arrangements were made to assure that treatment of the correct knee was carried out, and support for postoperative recovery was arranged. The fact that the surgeon had an excellent relationship with the patient was a factor in our favor. We notified the Department of Health.

A root-cause analysis was assembled. For unclear reasons, and despite the surgeon's appropriately indicating which knee was to undergo the procedure by "signing" the correct knee (he had actually put his initials right on the knee that was meant to be operated on), the contralateral limb was prepped and draped. The room had been set up differently than usual due to equipment-availability issues. A resident had placed purple marks on the now-draped knee to show scope-insertion sites. The checklist was run, and on the segment "site and side confirmed" team members compared the consent and operative schedule. A few glanced at the leg and saw some purple but couldn't say that they confirmed the surgeon's mark. A traveling nurse who was new to the time-out procedures was in the room. She had not been formally oriented as to the procedures. The surgeon was a superb technician but was quick to show displeasure with inefficiencies. Finally, the incorrect knee also had arthritic changes, which is what the surgeon had expected to see, leading to the delayed recognition of the problem. It was a classic error chain.

I spent a great deal of time trying to understand what went wrong. I thought we had a strong culture because the checklists were being used and people appeared to be talking to each other. Yet I learned that ambiguity existed as to what "site and side confirmed" meant. Parts of the checklist added little value and reduced the credibility of the process. New members of the team may not have been briefed on expectations or have felt comfortable speaking up.

Because of the high national visibility already focused on Rhode Island, the Department of Health was very active in the investigation of both the institution and individuals. Fortunately, we had been seen as proactive in patient safety initiatives, and the investigation sought to find solutions as opposed to finding someone to punish. Perhaps the strongest signal was sent when I was asked to appear before the Board of Licensure and Discipline to explain how this could happen. The question before me focused on whether the surgeon, as "captain of the ship," was ultimately responsible. In the past, it was the surgeon who would be censured. I said that we were all responsible, myself included.

The subsequent response was consistent with the just culture to which we aspire. The DOH sent a strong message by peer reviewing all the members of the surgical team. There was no licensing action, but the findings were made public.

In lieu of formal sanctions, everyone participated actively in fixing the problem and, more important, sharing with others their experiences. Steps in the checklists were clarified. For my part, I led a statewide initiative to standardize the Universal Protocol to minimize the possibility that a surgeon, who might work in multiple hospitals, would have to remember disparate marking and time-out protocols. Rhode Island committed to a statewide patient safety organization with mechanisms for sharing best practices, near misses, and areas of vulnerabilities.

Checklists and training reduce risk, but they are no guarantee that the team will function properly. That is our ongoing challenge.

At my new institution, Cedars-Sinai in Los Angeles, I'm involved in an initiative to prevent wrong-site surgery. When we reviewed our own experiences, patterns emerged that were similar to what I experienced in Rhode Island. Team dynamics often played a role. Various components of the marking protocols were inconsistently applied, and the dynamics of power and hierarchy were obvious. We educated, cajoled, and threatened. I was becoming somewhat discouraged.

A month ago, the holes in the Swiss cheese were about to line up one more time. An incorrect limb had been prepped, and the surgeon was sure he had marked the patient correctly. As a final check, one of the nurses picked up a discrepancy between the history and physical, consent, and X-rays. She spoke up and stopped the case before the incision.

We widely publicized her as the Safety Star of the Week in our harm report. The pride she felt being a patient advocate was supplemented by awarding her a prime parking space on the hospital campus here in West Hollywood.

And if that doesn't change behavior, I don't know what will.

• • •

HARRY C. SAX, MD is Professor and Executive Vice Chair of Surgery at Cedars-Sinai Medical Center in Los Angeles. He is actively involved in safety, quality, and team-building initiatives, both locally and nationally. Drawing on his experience as a general aviation pilot, he was one of the early advocates for the adoption of crew resource management techniques and checklists in medicine. He served as Chief Medical Officer at Hospital Sacre Coeur in Milot, Haiti, during recovery efforts after the 2010 earthquake.

Teaching a New Physician

Adam Elliott

I work as a registered nurse on an acute care neurosurgery unit in a teaching hospital; I've been there for just over three years. The RNs on my unit teach not only new nurses but also physicians-in-training, and that helps us all function as a team. Consider, for example, what happened recently when I came on shift to work a three-day weekend.

As I received my assignment of five patients with either brain or spinal cord injuries, I realized that I was the senior RN on the floor with two novice RNs working with me. Thankfully, they were wise beyond their years. Also working with us was a brand-new resident who had never worked on a neurosurgery unit before. In addition to my own patient load, I was in charge of the seventeen-bed ward while mentoring the new RN staff and our new resident. Our typical patients, either brain- or spinal cord–injured people, can be pre-op, post-op, or have tumors that require removal. These patients are considered acute and unstable and require complex medication regimens, as well as intense physiotherapy (in cases where loss of function or paralysis may have occurred). Our floor has, thus, developed a very holistic team-centered approach.

In the middle of rounds on Saturday, I was explaining to our medical resident how to correctly adjust Phenytoin dosages, a medication we use on our floor to help keep patients from seizing and further injuring their brains. (Dosage is determined by a calculation of various blood levels within the body, as the drug binds with some of the body's natural chemicals.) Suddenly, we heard a shout from a room down the hall: "I'm going to need a hand! Seizure!" The resident and I went to see what was going on and found a patient in a four-bed ward room having a violent grand mal seizure and the RN initiating seizure protocol—which includes various measures to protect the patient's airway (suctioning any sputum, administering oxygen, and turning him to his side to keep the airway open), as well as giving him Lorazepam (a drug that helps stop a seizure) and checking his vital signs.

The other three patients in the room were looking on in horror, as was our resident. The assigned RN and I helped the man through his seizure and took some blood to check the Phenytoin levels to ensure that he was taking the correct dosage; after two-and-a-half long minutes, he finally stopped seizing. Our resident then slowly approached and asked if the patient was going to be okay. I told him that he'd been showing signs of increased intracranial pressure (a slower pulse rate, widening pulse pressure, confusion, nausea) and that he might have some swelling or he could be rebleeding from the surgery he had two days earlier. We suggested that he should order a repeat CT and adjust the patient's antiseizure and steroid dosages.

I had barely finished our sentence when the patient started to seize once again. We then immediately hung Dexamethasone and Mannitol to help bring down any further intracranial swelling. After he was given 300 mg of Mannitol, the patient finally began to perk up and become responsive once again. We then checked his Phenytoin levels and discovered that they were indeed low and that he needed an additional boost of the drug. After completing all of this, the assigned RN and I explained everything we'd done to the resident, who thanked us and ordered the immediate CT as requested. Throughout all of this, there were sixteen other patients on the floor to whom we were expected to provide the same care but who were left with just one junior RN while the other two of us were dealing with this situation.

I then went back to rounds with our doctor and checked my patients' vital signs. The doctor and I came to one patient whose Dexamethasone required adjusting. Since the resident had never ordered this drug prior to the previous episode, I explained how to taper the dose so the patient would experience the least amount of adverse effects.

After rounds were completed, the CT lab technician called for the patient who had been seizing earlier in the day. The other RNs on the floor were face-and-eyes into their morning work at this point, so I told the resident we now had a lovely learning opportunity here—secretly, I didn't want to bring this very acutely ill patient to CT alone, and at least the resident knew first aid—and that we should bring the patient down to do the RN a favor. He reluctantly agreed. I gathered the required supplies for portable seizure precautions (portable suction, oxygen, Lorazepam), and we took the patient to the lab. Thankfully, we got there safely and back upstairs to our unit. I then left the resident to review the CT and asked him to call the neurosurgery staff physician to get his opinion so that I could complete the work for the patients whom I hadn't seen since early morning.

The other RNs on the floor had just about finished their work for the day, so we all got together and completed mine. I had never been so grateful for the team approach on our unit. Thankfully, all of my patients were relatively healthy that day.

As it happened, the CT scan showed he had another bleed and thus he needed to be rushed to surgery that afternoon. Again, the other RNs and I got together to prep the patient for emergency surgery, administering IV fluids, steroids, putting on antithrobolytic stockings (to help keep him from developing blood clots during surgery) for the operating room, and doing other general work to prepare him for surgery, including calling the operating room to confirm a time, walking the new resident through the OR checklist, and gaining consents. Then we sent the patient off and anxiously awaited the outcome, hoping for positive results.

The patient arrived back from surgery a few hours later, groggy and sedated but dramatically improved. We all breathed a huge sigh of relief and felt good knowing that it was our assessment and critical intervention skills that likely saved his life. And we all felt good knowing that we had one another to depend on. Our new resident was also very thankful that we shared our knowledge with him and were able to intervene when he was essentially a spectator. He told us how relieved he was that we knew what we were doing. We laughed, told him it was all in a day's work, and said that Sunday morning coffee was on him.

· · ·

ADAM ELLIOTT, RN is a Registered Nurse on a Neurosurgical Unit in Newfoundland and Labrador and is working on his Masters of Nursing. Acknowledging the value of RNs in health care delivery, he is very engaged with the Newfoundland and Labrador Nurses Union (NLNU) and representing in RNs across his province and throughout Canada.

Teamwork and Perseverance Prevail

Fredrick B. Cassera

In many hospitals, pharmacies are located in the basement of the institution, which gives the pharmacists who work in them limited access—and limited visibility—to patients and physicians. Although most patients in the hospital receive multiple medications, and every new medication ordered must be reviewed by a pharmacist for therapeutic appropriateness, the value of the pharmacist as a member of the health care team is often overlooked.

In our hospital, pharmacists take an active role as part of the interdisciplinary clinical team that provides service to the patient, and our pharmacists are actually also on the units interacting directly with patients, families, and other health care team members. This approach, which is the optimal model, offers patients and health care providers immediate access to the knowledge and expertise that pharmacists are readily able and qualified to provide.

In our model of care, the inclusion of the pharmacist on the unit has resulted in positive outcomes that would not have occurred in a more traditional setting in which the pharmacist always remains out of sight and contact in the proverbial basement of the hospital. This story illustrates what can happen when pharmacists are truly integrated into the team.

On this particular day, an elderly male patient was admitted to the hospital, and the medical resident took the patient's medication history and entered it into his chart. As in most institutions, this history included a complete list of the medications the patient was taking at home, which is usually obtained directly from the patient, a family member, or from a list or perhaps prescription bottles that the patient is asked to bring to the hospital. This important safety check is always a challenge, particularly when the patient is on multiple medications, if there are language barriers, pronunciation difficulties, or slight memory issues. In this case, the patient did not speak English.

One of the medications on the patient's list was an estrogen modulator, a medication usually indicated for women for the prevention of osteoporosis or invasive breast cancer. This patient, however, was male. Since medications are routinely prescribed outside of FDA-approved indications, Paul, the clinical pharmacist who was assigned to the patient, knew that it was possible that a male might be prescribed an estrogen modulator for some legitimate clinical reason. However, when reviewing the order, Paul wanted to verify that it was prescribed as intended—rather than being a mistake. So he began a review of clinical references available to pharmacists practicing in the hospital. He also consulted with another clinical pharmacist. Both questioned the lack of good clinical evidence to support the use of this medication for this patient.

Paul then visited the patient to review and discuss the patient's medication history. Since the patient did not speak English, the family assisted and provided Paul with the prescription bottle from the community pharmacy. Indeed, it was clear that the patient was receiving the medication at home.

In most cases, the story would have ended right here. In the mind of an inquisitive clinical pharmacist, however, what he learned just wasn't good enough. Paul proceeded to contact the physician caring for the patient in the hospital. When Paul brought his concern about the indication for using the medication to the physician's attention, the resident paused and reflected. On the patient's admission to the hospital, the resident had dutifully checked the medications that had been brought from home and had copied the estrogen modulator in the medication profile. When Paul questioned him, however, he gave it a much-needed second thought and agreed that this was indeed an unusual order that required further investigation, which he asked Paul to pursue.

Paul contacted the community pharmacy that filled the original prescription. When this prescription was brought to the attention of the community pharmacist he too took a second look. It turned out that the prescription had been delivered to the community pharmacy via an e-prescription. The e-prescription is a relatively new mechanism that permits a physician to fill out a prescription electronically and transmit it to the pharmacy via the internet or fax.

This newer technology is intended to reduce the possibility of prescribing errors.

When the community pharmacist had received that prescription he thought that the medication might have been inappropriate. However, he figured that, since the medication order was generated by a computer technology touted for diminishing the likelihood of a medication error, the order was correct. Like many of us who believe in the power of technology, the community pharmacist felt sure the computer would have caught the mistake.

Prompted by Paul, the community pharmacist acknowledged that clarification of the order should be followed back to the prescribing physician to verify that this older man should really be receiving an estrogen modulator. Paul then contacted the physician who originally prescribed the medication, and he was equally concerned and surprised. "Why would I give an estrogen modulator to a male patient?" he asked.

He then referred Paul back to the community pharmacy where he believed the error must have occurred. Once again, Paul went the extra mile. He contacted the community pharmacist who reiterated that he had received the Rx via an e-prescription. The conscientious community pharmacist then also called the physician because he was concerned that he had received a prescription that the doctor said he'd never sent.

Soon afterward, the physician called Paul and said, "Look I treat both the husband and wife, and the error must have occurred when the e-prescription was sent for the husband rather than the wife." The physician thanked Paul and the community pharmacist for bringing this error to his attention. The medication was immediately discontinued. The private physician proceeded to electronically transmit a new prescription to the community pharmacy, this time intended for the patient's wife. The patient and family were informed of the medication error and were grateful that it was caught and resolved, particularly because the wife, who hadn't being getting her much-needed medication for osteoporosis for months, was now finally receiving it.

Listening to this story, one might wonder why the wife, who wasn't getting her medication for her osteoporosis, didn't question the physician. Or why the husband, who might have been having unwanted side effects from his wife's medication, didn't inquire why he was given a medication for no known reason. The fact is patients—all too often—are on multiple medications and are unlikely to challenge a physician about their medication regimens.

It's not uncommon for patients to respond to a question about a medication with, "Oh, I don't know what it's for; I just take that little pink pill twice a day." It's also not unusual for busy pharmacists in the community or residents in hospitals to dampen their curiosity because "the computer doesn't make mistakes" or because another physician has ordered the medication.

This is why the pharmacist's role on the team is such a critical one. This is what we are taught to think about and what we pay attention to. A pharmacist's participation and input is especially important today in a health care environment where people are rushed, frequently overworked, often fatigued, and sometimes have the unwarranted belief that physicians don't make errors or that the computers designed to prevent them always do their job. In this case, as in so many others, the resolution of this medication error occurred because of the perseverance of a committed member of the health care team who challenged conventional safeguards and wisdom and left no stone unturned. Good communication, committed cooperation, determination, and having the confidence to challenge technology enhanced the care received by both the patient and his wife. It should be noted that a month later Paul received our pharmacy's Best Catch Award for the most significant clinical intervention of the month.

· · ·

FREDRICK B. CASSERA, RPh, MS, MBA is Vice President of Pharmaceutical Services, Maimonides Medical Center in Brooklyn, New York. He is a clinical associate professor of pharmacy and a clinical preceptor in the experiential education component of pharmacy curriculum at St. John's University College of Pharmacy. He is chairman of the Pharmacy Advisory Committee for Greater New York Hospital Association and past president of the Royal Counties of New York Society of Hospital Pharmacists.

The Story of Our Patient Safety Fellows

Kathleen Burke

When we discuss teams in health care, we often think about people in different professions or occupations working together, communicating with one another as they share perspectives and information. In a system as complex as a large teaching hospital, like the one I work in, however, teamwork needs to exist not only among professions but within them. A profession like nursing does not always provide individual nurses from different departments or specialties with a mechanism to share with and learn from one another. For this reason, inside their own discipline, nurses may not always function as a collaborative team that works effectively across an institution or even on a particular unit or service.

At the University of California, San Francisco (UCSF) Medical Center, an effort to address and remedy this problem was launched in 2001 and has been ongoing ever since. The goal of this project, known as the UCSF Patient Safety Fellows, has been to identify critical safety issues that emerge in our daily work, share safety information and awareness of safety problems with all the nurses who work at UCSF, and share with nurses in the institution the insights and solutions that RNs have developed as they care for patients. This process hardwires the kind of institutional learning that is the foundation of a culture of safety.

The Patient Safety Fellows project began with a grant proposal written by two nurses at UCSF—Michael Fox, who was at the time a perinatal nurse, and Ann Williamson, who was the assistant director of nursing. The grant was funded by the University Health Consortium (a consortium of university-based hospitals, of which UCSF is a member, that collaborates on projects and creates benchmarks). The grant established a group of nurse "fellows" at UCSF and sent them to Dayton, Ohio, to train with Klein Associates. Gary Klein has developed a training focused on certain debriefing skills that have been identified as crucial for effective team communication, analysis of decision making, and root-cause analysis of errors.

Through Klein's methods, a bedside nurse who is neither a nurse manager nor in an administrative position can learn the kind of debriefing skills that would allow him or her to sit down with another bedside nurse and debrief an incident of patient harm or error or near miss. As many of us have learned the hard way, unraveling a problem or figuring out why an error occurred isn't so easy. When you ask questions in the wrong way people become defensive and conceal rather than reveal. If you don't ask the right questions or probe deeply enough, you won't learn about the complex circumstances that led to the error. On the surface, some of these circumstances may not appear to be relevant to the error or incident, but they may have actually played a significant role in the event.

Klein's trainings teach people what questions to ask and how to ask them. It also teaches us how to create a neutral environment that allows questions to be raised in a way that doesn't produce a biased answer or that sacrifices pertinent information.

The goal of the debriefing is to deconstruct the event so that a fuller picture of what actually happened emerges. This information is then shared with other nurses to collectively learn from that incident, mistake, or error.

After going to Ohio, Fox and Williamson and six of their colleagues came back to UCSF and began to solicit case scenarios so they could present them in a group setting that would encourage shared learning. The Patient Safety Fellows, who began to meet once a month, would solicit stories that could be debriefed and decided which ones to present at a series of larger classes that became known as Stories from the Bedside. Initially, to become a Patient Safety Fellow, a nurse would apply for the fellowship and had to satisfy some fairly stringent requirements—such as attending a certain number of monthly meetings or going to an application interview. The group quickly decided that this process erected too many barriers to participation and so we created a fairly informal process for participation in the group. Nurses could simply come to a monthly Patient Safety Fellows meeting and express interest in building a better safety culture at UCSF.

Once the grant money for training was exhausted, the Patient Safety Fellows program continued with the support of the Department of Nursing. Over the past ten years, fellows have continued to meet for two hours on a monthly basis and hold Stories from the Bedside classes four times a year. We have also added a communication skills class, Life Saving Skills for Nurses: Effective Communication for Patient Safety, which has been given twice a year. Although we often think of life saving skills as CPR or electric shock, in fact, the number one cause of sentinel events in hospitals is failure in communication. In the class, we provide nurses with skills on how to communicate effectively when critical information has to be exchanged in routine, stressful, or urgent situations.

Any nurse in our institution is invited to attend the Stories classes, and nurses receive continuing education units for their participation. Nurses are able to use education time to attend the sessions, which last four hours each. We usually get between thirty and ninety nurses at each session. The stories that are shared and analyzed in these sessions are gathered in the monthly meetings of the Patient Safety Fellows.

During these meetings, nurses share safety concerns that they have either observed or been made aware of or that stem from incidents they themselves have experienced. Stories typically begin with, "You know what happened on my unit?" Listening to the narrative, we often realize that similar things are happening in one form or another throughout the institution. The stories thus reveal larger system or procedural deficiencies. If closeted within a particular unit or one individual's ruminations, there can be no recognition that there is a broader problem and therefore no mechanism for situational awareness, change, or improvement.

We then decide which particular story is important enough to bring to the attention of a larger group. If we uncover an urgent problem, we will report it to nursing administration to alert them. For example, a nurse alerted us to the fact that RNs on her unit were overriding the IV pump safety programming because the volume of fluid in certain antibiotic IV bags was not matching the programmed volume in the smart pumps. Those of us who have safety awareness recognized that anytime a nurse has to override the programmed smart pump (which is considered a work-around) it creates an opportunity for error or harm to patients. We went to the assistant director of nursing with this problem, and she subsequently made sure that pediatric nursing administration and the director of the pediatric pharmacy got together to discuss and remedy it. The nurse who reported the problem was also involved in designing and implementing its solution.

Like so many other issues that we analyze, this one was a case of everyone knowing there was a problem yet dealing with it through work-arounds or what Tucker and Edmondson call "first-order thinking."[6] Once the Patient Safety Fellows collectively identified it as a problem that needed resolution sooner rather than later, the tendency to normalize the work-around on the unit was challenged and the problem was solved on a system-wide basis.

Stories that do not need urgent attention are presented at formal Stories at the Bedside sessions. The stories we pick represent a good learning opportunity for other nurses. Before the formal presentation, the Patient Safety Fellows discuss the story among ourselves and analyze the risks it presents for either patients or safe nursing practice. We then pick a theme around this primary case and look for other stories or cases that include similar themes. In this way, we determine the focus of that particular session.

We invite the nurse who brought us the case to present it to the entire group. Before his or her formal presentation, we coach that nurse about how to recount the story in a way that peels back the layers of the onion to make visible the thinking, actions, decisions, or circumstances that set the patient up for harm or error. We give the nurses templates that help them tell their story in a way that illuminates the decision points and communication issues or system failures that led to the problem. Our hope is that through these examples, nurses learn that there are resources, insights, new skills, or research that could help them better prevent this same error.

Once nurses are prepared for the formal sessions, a facilitator for each class begins that four-hour class by discussing the context and safety themes that the stories spotlight—for example, the global problem of errors during medication administration and the nurse's role in minimizing them. The facilitator also leads the discussion that follows the story presentation. During that discussion the facilitator is careful to tease out general safety concepts around effective communication, situational awareness, why a policy is in place and should be followed, and good cross monitoring and to end with lessons learned.

In one recent class, for example, a pediatric nurse told the following story. Baby Jane was ordered to receive 3 mcg of digoxin elixir. The dose received from the pharmacy was labeled with the correct concentration of 0.05 mg per ml, which, if calculated 3 micrograms would be 0.06 ml. The syringe provided by the pharmacy to the floor contained 0.6 mls, which at that concentration equals 30, not 3, mcg. So, if administered with that syringe, Baby Jane would have gotten ten times the ordered dose. As per policy, a second RN checked the order and syringe and questioned the volume amount in the syringe. This revealed the potential error. Pharmacy was contacted, and a new syringe with the proper amount of medication was delivered to the unit. The take-away message here was that an accurate, independent check by a second RN is critical to safe medication administration—which is why we must follow policy.

A lay person hearing this story might respond with shock that this message needs to be reiterated. But, in the real world of a hospital, there are so many interruptions and so much stress that lessons must be repeated over and over again, and nurses must be reminded of the consequences of their diligence and vigilance to details—even to those they seemingly have no control over. In this case, it was the pharmacist who put the incorrect volume in the syringe, but it was the nurses who caught the error. In medication administration, no matter who writes the order or fills the prescription, when it comes down to the nurse administering the medication to the patient, that RN is the final check between safety and harm. Of course, we have a twenty-eight-page nursing medication administration policy. Having nurses read this policy is not what's going to guarantee that the right patient gets the right medication at the right dose via the right route at the right time. When nurses sitting in the audience hear stories from other working nurses, their emotional response to real cases and their collective and individual reflection on their own nursing practice can create the "aha!" moments that help us all understand why what's in that twenty-eight-page policy statement is important.

The patient safety physician Donald Berwick has commented that "the will for change [to safety culture] in a complex system like [health care] comes from narrative, not from numbers." Over the last decade our Patient Safety Fellows have tried to move beyond the numbers and abstractions by using real examples unique to our medical center to bring home the message that it happens here on our own units. By learning what discrete individuals have done in particular situations, we create institutional models of safety and lay the foundation for a broader safety culture.

More than this, the process of engaging in collective reflection— both in our monthly meetings and our Stories classes—presents an opportunity for nurses from the same institution but who practice in different areas to recognize that they are, in fact, part of a team. As a high-functioning team, they debrief together and learn from one another so that they can leave a session with new insights and safety awareness. They can thus enhance their own individual practice and help create new situational and safety awareness on their units and throughout the institution.

· · ·

KATHLEEN BURKE, RN is a staff nurse at University of California, San Francisco Medical Center. She is Co-Chair of the UCSF Patient Safety Fellows Committee. In 2007, she was recognized for Excellence in Patient Safety from the UCSF Department of Nursing.

The Inconvenience of Safety

Handel Reynolds

I had received ample forewarning. My first afternoon patient was a woman returning to have a breast biopsy redone, and she was decidedly annoyed at the prospect. The patient was a busy forty-six year old who spent her days managing a large sporting goods store and her evenings managing two teenage sons whom she was raising alone. She was a very intense woman for whom the loss of control that comes with being a patient was a wholly unnatural experience. In her world, she called the shots. She had no tolerance for inept people or ineffectual systems. She had recently received the news that the lump she had found in her left breast was malignant. To add insult to injury, the breast magnetic resonance imaging scan her surgeon ordered following her diagnosis revealed an unsuspected suspicious mass in the right breast. An MRI is often performed on newly diagnosed breast cancer patients. This highly sensitive test not only gives a very detailed rendition of the known tumor, including its size and relationship to other anatomical structures, but in about 15 percent of cases, an additional breast cancer is found in the diseased breast, and in about 3 percent of cases, an unsuspected cancer is found in the opposite breast.

She had been in our breast center the week before to have a biopsy of the unsuspected right breast mass that the MRI had disclosed. However, due to an equipment failure during the procedure, the biopsy could not be completed. She had spent two hours of her overtaxed life in this, ultimately futile, attempt to get answers.

I met the patient for the first time on the afternoon of the second biopsy attempt. Even though she had been in this very position just days earlier, it was necessary for me to review the details of the procedure with her. I had not been involved in the previous episode, and she would have to give her informed consent for me to proceed. I informed her of the steps that had been taken to ensure that the technical difficulties encountered last time would not recur. Not surprisingly, she seemed irritated at the whole situation and very eager to "get it over with."

The Joint Commission requires a preprocedure pause, or time-out protocol, immediately prior to the initiation of any invasive procedure. This protocol calls for a three-point confirmation: correct patient, correct procedure, and correct site. The patient's identity is confirmed by referring to her identification wristband. The procedure and site are verified by referring to the physician's order. In performing this preprocedure pause, we discovered that the order her surgeon had provided simply stated "image-guided breast biopsy." The site (right breast) was not specified.

Even though she knew the procedure was to be performed on her right breast, and the entire procedure team did as well, the biopsy could not begin until a fully compliant physician's order was in hand. The most expeditious way to accomplish this would be for me to speak with her surgeon and have her instruct her office to immediately fax me a new order. I called the surgeon's office. She was in a procedure room with a patient. After I waited on hold for about ten to fifteen minutes, she came to the phone and I apprised her of the situation. She confirmed that it was the right breast that was to be biopsied and promptly provided a new order that specified the site. When I returned to the holding room where the patient was waiting, her mood, which had not been pleasant to begin with, had noticeably soured. Irritation had given way to pure disgust—a state of mind that she made no attempt to disguise. Though unspoken, the urgency of the moment was fully grasped by the team. We performed the time-out procedure and completed the biopsy without further incident.

A few days following the biopsy, I received a letter from the patient. It was not one of those letters thanking the "whole staff for their outstanding care" that we so enjoy receiving. Rather, this was a particularly angry letter in which she painstakingly detailed her displeasure with the service she received at her last visit. The delay caused by the issue with the physician's order had, among other things, caused her to miss a very important meeting at her older son's school. She would have to take time off, yet again, to attend to this matter. She saw no reason that we could not have proceeded with the biopsy since everyone involved already knew which breast was to be biopsied.

"Was the patient's time and her family and work commitments not more important than a clerical technicality?" she demanded.

In my reply I apologized for the inconvenience and stress she had endured but also tried to explain to her the principles of safety we endeavor to adhere to with every patient. I tried to reassure her that the time taken to confer with her surgeon was an essential step in building a safety shield around her, a barrier that hopefully would lessen the likelihood of an undesirable outcome.

I never heard back from her. I later learned that she had been successfully treated and had fully resumed her superbusy life. This experience was an important one for me because it opened my eyes to a dynamic that I had not previously contemplated. That is, the tension between safety and efficiency. In the twenty-first century, patients, rightly or wrongly, tend to *assume* safety and earnestly *hope for* efficiency. Time-out protocols and obsession over paperwork, with all the right boxes checked, can sometimes seem like pointless speed bumps in our modern fast-paced existence. Deep in our hearts many of us harbor the idealistic notion that in today's technologically advanced medical environment, the chance of the wrong procedure being done is practically zero. We step into the health care world *expecting* everything to be done right. Physicians almost never receive letters thanking them for the lack of complications or other mishaps. At the same time, they frequently receive letters thanking them for compassionate care and *efficiently rendered* services. Safety is expected. There are no special accolades when that standard is met. Efficiency is a variable, a highly subjective measure that has a powerful impact on patient satisfaction. Carefully balancing these two metrics is essential to achieving success in health care.

· · ·

The late HANDEL REYNOLDS, MD, FACR was a breast radiologist in private practice and at the Doris Shaheen Breast Health Center at Piedmont Hospital in Atlanta, Georgia. He was formerly Associate Professor of Radiology and Chief of Breast Radiology at Indiana University. He wrote *The Big Squeeze: A Social and Political History of the Controversial Mammogram* (Ithaca: Cornell University Press, 2012).

Do You Feel Like a Caregiver?

K. Kelly Hancock and James I. Merlino

"Do you feel like a caregiver?" K. Kelly Hancock, the Cleveland Clinic's executive chief nursing officer, asked a group of security staff at the Cleveland Clinic. There was a short awkward silence, and then "Yes, we do!" was the reply. "We have been talking about this caregiver thing for over four years now. Do you really feel part of the team—like you are involved in helping to take care of patients, just like everyone else across the street?" asked Dr. James I. Merlino, chief experience officer. The group gave an overwhelming response: "Absolutely!" They felt like they were a big part of the mission at Cleveland Clinic and were essential to the care of patients.

We were spending time talking to the Cleveland Clinic's Police Department's morning roll call. We had been rounding on different groups across the clinic, and we were now determined to hit all three roll calls throughout the day. Hancock's question was spontaneous. We knew that the police were essential to the mission of the clinic, but we were curious if they actually felt a connection to the rest of the organization as true caregivers.

When Dr. Delos "Toby" Cosgrove became CEO of Cleveland Clinic, he introduced the motto "Patients first." He really wanted to send the message that the only reason the organization exists is to care for patients and that everyone in the organization needed to revolve around the patient. Wanting to take the organization even further, he identified everyone as a caregiver. He wanted the organization to break down the silos of rank and reinforce the fact that medicine is a team sport. It did not matter if you were a surgeon or a maintenance worker in the basement making sure the lights came on in the morning; if you worked for Cleveland Clinic, you were responsible for supporting the mission, which is to provide world-class care to patients. This was a tough change for people to accept. Some physicians believed that if you were not a nurse or a doctor there was no way you could be a caregiver or have anything particularly insightful to contribute. Similarly, some nonmedical people, who had no patient contact, had a hard time understanding how they were caregivers.

The "caregiver" label was not intended to be just a marketing ploy. To cement that it had real meaning, the clinic leadership designed an exercise called the Cleveland Clinic Experience. All employees—including physicians—were required to attend. Employees were randomly assigned to sit around a table of eight to ten people. Physicians found themselves sitting next to nurses or maintenance staff or pharmacists, and for three and a half hours, all these various kinds of "caregivers" had conversations about why it is important to put patients first; how we are all in this together as a team—that is, we are all caregivers; the importance of service excellence; and how the organization's values contribute to our work. It took a year to put 43,000 people through this experience, but after the exercise the clinic saw its highest rise in patient-experience and employee-engagement scores and the steepest decline in patient complaints.

At the morning report we attended and at the two subsequent shift changes, we asked the police officers if they had ideas that would improve patient care. They did, and they offered many ideas that were well thought out and that targeted important issues. They saw aspects of the organization that no one else sees and helped us understand many technical problems that were frustrating to patients.

The Cleveland Clinic encompasses twenty-nine blocks, with multiple areas for patient care spread across the campus. One officer pointed out that the information patients receive about directions to the campus lists the main clinic address. When patients put this address into their GPS devices, they all end up at the main entrance, which in most cases is nowhere near where their appointment is located. This causes significant congestion and subsequent patient and family dissatisfaction. Another officer commented that at routine discharge times, the main entrance was cluttered, and often family members had to wait in their cars for up to an hour to get near the door to pick up a discharged patient. This observation even came with a solution: "Have patients discharged around the corner at the side entrance to relieve the main entrance congestion—there is more room and easier vehicle access." We would never have thought of that.

Officers from all of the shifts talked about the need for more benches so patients can take breaks when walking across the large campus. Others described how they are occasionally called to assist on the nursing floors with an angry family member. They went on to describe that in their experience, if the floor caregivers had done a better job in diffusing the situation, perhaps the police would not have needed to be called. One said, "There is nothing worse than having a family member addressed by the police when they are already experiencing one of their worst moments." They suggested that the police calls to the floors be regularly reviewed and requested that they participate in staff debriefings. All of their suggestions were distributed to the appropriate operations areas for review and implementation. Every suggestion is being evaluated, and several are already being implemented. The department that manages hospital discharges is changing how patients are discharged; we are updating our patient communications to better assist in giving accurate directions; and we are reviewing all calls involving the police being sent to the nursing floors. The police suggestions were invaluable in helping us to take better care of our patients and our people.

The police had not only adopted the "caregiver" label but also they were actively involved in seeking ways to improve our patients' experience. We were frankly floored by the level of engagement from our police force—and we told them so. One officer finally remarked, "Sometimes we feel that people forget about us, that they don't believe we are part of the team, and we get left out of things like recognition events." We aim for that never to happen again.

• • •

K. KELLY HANCOCK, RN is Executive Chief Nursing Officer, Cleveland Clinic health system and Chief Nursing Officer, Main Campus. Previously, she served as the Chief Nursing Officer at Main Campus. She has simultaneously been the Senior Nursing Director of Critical Care and the Nursing Director of the Heart and Vascular Institute, where she led the nursing practice in the Heart and Vascular Institute for seven years.

JAMES I. MERLINO, MD is the Chief Experience Officer and Associate Chief of Staff of the Cleveland Clinic health system. He is also a practicing colorectal surgeon in the Digestive Disease Institute and founder and president of the Association for Patient Experience. In addition to his work in patient experience, he leads efforts to improve physician-patient communication, patient access, and referring-physician relations. He is a recognized world leader in the emerging field of patient experience.

I'm Not Sorry for Calling You

Paulina Bleah

The nurse-doctor relationship has always been a tricky phenomenon to me, partly because I never understood why there was so much animosity and competition between nurses and doctors and also because of my inclination as a nurse to feel inferior to physicians. I believe that as a student, during my clinical experience, I was socialized to "shut up, listen, and do." I was timid, obedient, and never challenged the status quo. After graduation, I began working in an acute medical unit where everything was rush-rush and go-go. Again, the importance of following doctors' orders was reinforced. In this setting, nurse managers and physicians placed a great deal of emphasis on understanding the value of their time—that is, physicians' time. Point blank, nurses were not to call a doctor unless it was a "life or death" matter, as one attending physician put it.

For many months, I worked within this system and was careful not to call the doctor unless one of my patients was at such great risk that neither I nor members of my nursing team could handle the situation. I observed nurses always cautioning one another when making decisions about whether to dial the doctor. When nurses did call the doctor, they often started the conversation with an apology and then proceeded to state their request. Initially, I never questioned this practice and also found myself doing the same thing. It was the culture; I did not dare to challenge it.

A year into my practice, I had an epiphany. I was working a night shift, and about three hours into my shift, I sat down to do some charting as my patients were settled in bed. While sitting at the nursing station, I overheard one of my nursing colleagues on the phone speaking with a doctor. She was calling about a concern she had for one of her patients and wanted clarification. She started the conversation with the following, "Hello, I am so, so, so sorry to bother you, but I have concerns about my patient. Here are my concerns." She ended the conversation with, "Thank you and again I am really sorry for bothering you." The call started with an apology and ended with an apology. As I understand it, the purpose of an apology is to express regret for an offense. At that moment, for the first time in my nursing career I refused to let the status quo reign.

I approached the nurse and asked what she had done that was so terribly wrong that she was so apologetic.

Her response was "I don't know; it's just habit. Plus they are always so busy, I felt bad."

I responded, "But when you are busy, which is often the case, when the doctor calls you, does he apologize before making his demands?"

"No," she said.

"Then, why do you apologize for calling the doctor to inform him of serious concerns for your patient?" I asked.

She had no response and continued with her work.

That experience, that moment, challenged me. Later that night I said to my colleague, "No more. Don't apologize for calling the doctor."

· · ·

PAULINA BLEAH, BScN, RN is a staff nurse at Toronto General Hospital (TGH) on General Internal Medicine (GIM). She did her undergraduate at Ryerson University and is pursuing her masters in the Primary Health Care Nurse Practitioner Program at her alma mater. Bleah led a fellowship project, a quality improvement initiative on promoting urinary continence on GIM. In addition to her clinical work, Bleah annually travels to Liberia, West Africa, on mission trips and volunteers at hospitals, clinics, and orphanages. She was a fellow in the Collaborative Academic Practice Innovation and Research Fellowship Program at University Health Network (UHN).

Coaching the Huddle

Rebecca Shunk

In April 2010, as part of ongoing work on teamwork and interprofessional care at the Veterans Administration, as well as in response to the Affordable Care Act's focus on "medical homes" (a health care delivery model based on teams), a new team-based model of primary care was launched throughout the VA system. All primary care clinics in the VA nationwide are expected to launch Patient Aligned Care Teams (PACTs) that include primary care providers (physicians and nurse practitioners), registered nurses (RNs), licensed vocational nurses (LVNs), and clerks.

One critical part of this model is implementing what are known as "huddles." In the primary care clinic the huddle is a preclinic meeting where team members come together to review the schedule for the day, consider the needs of patients, troubleshoot problems, plan for upcoming visits, and discuss between-visit patient communications, which we refer to as telephone visits.

As a primary care provider and a leader in our clinic where we train new physicians, I was expected to help implement the huddle process. The problem was that although I had done significant reading on the topic of medical homes and knew about the existence of huddles, I knew very little about how to actually participate in a huddle. Implementing this team-based approach turned out to be much more involved than reading the literature or going to a seminar.

I remember the first day of huddling. I arrived at the clinic ready for my usual eight o'clock patient only to hear our team nurse say that my schedule had been changed, and we were going to huddle instead. We gathered in the assigned clinic room, looked at one another, and I asked, "Does anyone know exactly what we actually do in a huddle?" So began what turned out to be a rewarding adventure in team-based care.

Our learning curve as a team quickly accelerated when, several months later, our academic faculty team received a Center of Excellence (COE) award in Primary Care Education. The Office of Academic Affiliations in the VA provided $5 million to develop innovative ways to teach interprofessional trainees the key concepts of team-based patient-centered care. With the award we rapidly ramped up our education in the team-based model, moving beyond the concepts and into the tangible items such as developing a common language. Our practical training included an interprofessional group retreat to train in TeamSTEPPS. In all we sent over twenty people, including key RN and LVN staff, a chief resident, and psychologists, as well as a nurse practitioner (NP) and a physician (MD) who were faculty members. Ultimately, the VA delivered to all PACT teams a hands-on nuts-and-bolts training for two and a half days that accelerated our skills even further.

Nonetheless, in the early stages of our PACT, the huddles were not always happening, and when they did occur some providers and staff did not find them useful. This was primarily because people did not know the purpose of the huddle or their roles in it. When our first cohort of trainees arrived, we quickly realized that we needed to improve the functioning of the huddles—the key place where interprofessional trainees and staff communicate and collaborate.

We initially implemented a master huddle schedule and a huddle checklist. The checklist provided structure to the huddle, reminding all team members about the clinically meaningful components of the huddle. Key items are to review the patients of the day and their agendas; recent hospital charges; and complex patients who would benefit from seeing other members of the team such as those from behavioral health psychology, pharmacy, or social work. Although the huddle checklist did provide needed structure, it did not assure that the huddles actually happened or that all parts of the huddle occurred. We devised a plan to have the clinic preceptors of the day become huddle coaches. Our huddle coach program has made all the difference in helping our teams become high functioning.

Each interprofessional faculty member (NP and MD) was assigned a huddle. Huddle coach brainstorming sessions led by local experts in patient and team communication initially helped determine best practices for huddle coaches, as this was new to all of us. In the early stages of new huddles, the huddle coach simply made sure everyone attended the huddle. This commonly meant tracking down missing team members (trainee and staff) and reinforcing the importance of the huddles. Early on, coaches prioritized the need for a check-in so team members got to know one another personally and professionally, which fostered team cohesion. As team members gained more experience with the huddles and learned about each other, they began to find value in them, especially in how huddles assist in care coordination.

Once everyone was committed to attending the huddles, the coach moved on from confirming attendance to more advanced huddle coaching. Coaches began interjecting clinical content (how the trainee can treat hypothyroidism for example) and also clinic systems content (such as where patients can get their blood drawn). Arguably, the most important role the huddle coach plays is that of process observer. The huddle coach comments on team process, reminding the team, for example, that the RN does not schedule patients for the team; the clerk does. It also includes making sure all team members' voices are heard, including that of the clerk, NP student, or pharmacist. Team communication skills such as closed-loop communication and check-back are reinforced and noted when absent. Huddle coaches find that even seasoned teams occasionally require reinforcing for early-stage issues such as a check-in or timeliness. For the huddle coaches this simply reinforces their value to the team. Even though we've been doing this now for four years, huddle coach brainstorming sessions continue and help support our huddle coaches through peer-to-peer teaching and feedback.

Our huddle coaching program was initially designed to support the huddles for our Center of Excellence trainees. As a result of our coaching-trainee huddles, the staff in those huddles have taken what they have learned and have coached other huddles. The RN, LVN, and clerk staff are now the experts and act as informal coaches and active teachers of the new trainees when they arrive each year.

It is hard to describe the impact that team-based care has had on the clinic. Our huddle coaching program is a key part of developing these high-functioning teams. Skilled coaches praise collaborative care, point out communication lapses, and model nonhierarchical practice. Our high-functioning teams are best illustrated in the story of Maria, a clerk in our clinic. Although she has worked in our primary care clinic for many years, I am embarrassed to say I did not know her name prior to implementation of PACT. She has grown into her role as the clinic has become a true medical home. As her role in the huddle has been defined she has been given an important voice that makes a difference in the team.

I remember the day I realized we had truly changed the culture of our clinic. We were having our morning huddle when I asked Maria to cancel the appointment of a patient who had schizophrenia. Maria, who previously would not have spoken to me or challenged anything I had to say, asked me if I really thought it was a good idea to cancel him. She went on to elaborate. She told me she had to make three different phone calls to arrange for his visit and that scheduling the appointment I was about to cancel had required extensive cajoling. She added, "Do you remember he has trust issues? I am not sure he will ever come back if we cancel this appointment."

It was at that moment I realized the change we had made and that we had reached a critical point. Everyone had learned to work together, and we would never go back to our silos again. We all know now that working together we provide better care to our veterans.

· · ·

REBECCA SHUNK, MD is currently the physician Co-Director of the Center of Excellence in Primary Care Education at the San Francisco VA Medical Center. She is also the Associate Director of the PRIME Program as well as an Associate Professor at the University of California, San Francisco. The UCSF Teaching Scholars course further fostered her curriculum-development skills. Her work in developing a team-based model of ambulatory internal medicine residency training led her to her current role. She and her team innovate to develop strategies to improve interprofessional team-based health professions' education in patient-centered primary care.

Part 6

PATIENT ADVOCACY AS TEAM SPORT

Advocating effectively for patients and their families is an essential component of safe, high-quality care. But what precisely does it mean to be a "patient advocate" or to "advocate" for the patient? Look up the word in the dictionary and you find that advocate comes from the Latin *ad-vocare*. *Vocare* means "to call" and *ad* means "to"—so *advocare* means to call to (one's aid). Seek further and you find that an advocate is a person who publicly supports or recommends a particular cause or policy. Webster's defines an advocate as a defender of a cause or another person or as someone who speaks or writes to support something. The connection between advocacy and psychological safety could not be more clear. Because a person cannot advocate by thinking something and keeping it to oneself or wishing a patient well and hoping bad things don't happen, advocacy means taking some kind of public stand. This can take various forms, from the nurse who works hard to coordinate getting the right care to the bedside at the right time in the right way to the team that helps patients and their families navigate a very complex, fragmented care environment with multiple providers. Advocacy involves the outright refusal to leave patients to fend for themselves, because no one is connecting the pieces of the puzzle. We know that failure of advocacy not only leads to frustration but also to substandard care and even avoidable harm.[1]

Advocacy is particularly critical when it comes to teamwork and will become even more important given the current focus on the coordination of patient- and family-centered care. Building systems of care to make this easier so that it is the norm rather than the exception will be one of our most difficult challenges as we move forward.

One reason that advocacy is such a challenge is that it has been traditionally defined as an individual professional responsibility rather than as a team activity. In fact, advocacy is often used as a way that professionals and professions define themselves in opposition to one another. For over two decades, nurses, for example, have claimed that they are "the patient's advocate."[2] Imagine that statement in caps and italics. When physicians, social workers, or physical therapists hear that claim, they often respond, "So what does that make me, the patient's enemy?" In health care everyone seems to stake out ownership of the patient. What this section spotlights is what happens when the professions join together to advocate for the patient and just how powerful that collective advocacy can be.

In considering these stories, readers might be tempted to question caregivers' ability to apply such high standards to everyone who comes into their institution. These are exceptional cases, after all. Who has the time or resources to do this over and over again? If that's your first response, consider this. One of the beauties of teamwork is that the extraordinary can become the ordinary when people really work together. What dooms patients who have complex illnesses or problems to receiving only the most basic standard of care (if even that) is the failure to create and sustain the kind of genuine teams that make advocacy for higher standards a collective expectation and endeavor.

The Complex Discharge Needs of Mr. and Mrs. K

Chiara Campitelli-Thompson

It was just another admission on August 21, 2011, when Mr. K entered our specialized geriatrics rehabilitation unit at Providence Healthcare. At that time, I had no idea his case was going to be one of the most interesting, challenging, and collaborative cases of my eleven-year career as a social worker. It all began when our admitting department informed me and another social worker that Mrs. K was admitted following a stroke and Mr. K with "failure to cope" as a result of his wife's hospitalization. Mr. K was admitted to our geriatric rehabilitation unit and Mrs. K to our specialized stroke unit. We soon learned that these two patients were deeply intertwined in their decision making and did not have any other family or support system to assist with the discharge-planning process.

This was not the first time I had had a case with a husband and wife on two different units. For me, however, it was the first time our teams needed to work so closely together to ensure a safe discharge. Soon after the Ks were admitted, many interesting issues and challenges came to light. These included their codependent relationship, lack of social supports, an eviction notice owing to years of hoarding and unsafe clutter that resulted in a public health risk and condemnation of their apartment, a neglected and abused pet, refusal to follow team recommendations, lack of financial stability, and personality challenges that developed into barriers to proceeding with discharge plans.

Within our organization, interprofessional collaboration within and among units is common practice. Weekly, the unit doctor, assigned nurse, pharmacist, social worker, occupational therapist, physiotherapist, dietician, recreational therapist, and unit manager meet and hold interprofessional rounds. During these rounds, they discuss each patient in depth. In a round table or popcorn-style discussion each team member provides an update on the patient's progress as it relates to his or her rehabilitation goals and discharge. If there are any concerns, challenges, or barriers, these are also discussed.

Once we recognized the challenges involved in caring for Mr. and Mrs. K, the unit social workers made contact to schedule the meeting for both interprofessional teams to meet to discuss their concerns together. This allowed us to work collaboratively in problem solving and discharge planning.

In the first few weeks, the collaboration and teamwork involved many telephone conversations among the professionals involved in this case. Fifty-nine different staff members and community agency representatives were involved over the five months both patients were in our care. The professionals included the patient-flow coordinator, social workers, physiotherapists, occupational therapists, nurses, registered practical nurses, pharmacists, psychiatrists, patient care (unit) managers, senior management (director of nursing), rehabilitation assistants, dieticians, a unit volunteer, unit administrative assistants, in-house legal representatives, the Community Care Access Centre, in-house ethics specialists, unit physicians, a community health navigator, a public health nurse, their apartment superintendent and property manager, legal aid, the Advocacy Centre for the Elderly (ACE), the Landlord and Tenant Board, housing agencies, Scotia Bank, the Humane Society, and Revenue Canada.

Staff in these groups had to confirm and discuss assessment outcomes, obtain accurate details about the couple's living environment, and get information about caregiving roles and duties. In the weeks following, interprofessional consultation, problem solving, and partnership were required on a daily, weekly, and often on-the-go basis. This took place by way of e-mails, telephone and hallway conversations, joint assessments, joint team meetings, and brainstorming and strategy sessions with senior management and ethicists who facilitated in-depth deliberations.

The issue of their abused and neglected pet was a delicate one that came to light immediately after their admission to our care. Mrs. K had a unique attachment to her dog—she described it as her child. Over the years, if one dog died, Mrs. K always purchased the exact same breed and gave the dog the same name. Whenever one of the dogs died, she became very depressed and put the deceased animal in a basket and slept with it for many days. When Mr. and Mrs. K were hospitalized, a friend took in their pet to look after it and quickly came forward to the interprofessional teams to report its abuse. In almost four years, the animal had never been walked, never left their apartment, and never had contact with any other animals or people. The animal used the apartment as its latrine, and feces were matted to its fur. It had never seen a veterinarian. Its claws had grown so long that they curled underneath and into the bottom of its paws. The dog actually bled when it walked. Finally, it was so terrified of humans, it was incontinent and would attack or bite anyone who came near it.

The abuse needed to be reported to the Ontario Society for the Prevention of Cruelty to Animals (OSPCA). Because we knew how attached Mrs. K was to the dog and how she reacted when her last dog died, we, as an interprofessional team, worried about what impact reporting this abuse would have on her mental health. We also worried how such a drastic event would impact her poststroke recovery. Mr. K often made comments such as, "she will kill herself if anything happens to that dog."

After much deliberation and in-depth consultation, we all agreed the abuse had to be reported. One of the social workers made the telephone report, and the friend who was looking after the dog secretly took the animal to see a veterinarian. The veterinarian was devastated by the condition of the dog and had no choice but to euthanize it. However, Mr. and Mrs. K were not able to acknowledge that their pet had been abused or neglected and had seen nothing wrong with its condition—in fact, they completely denied it. We decided to tell Mrs. K that the animal had "passed away." The teams also decided to ask our psychiatrist to follow up with Mrs. K immediately after the animal's death and for her social worker to provide supportive counseling. Additionally, Mrs. K had connected deeply with one of her nurses who was an animal lover, so this nurse also provided a significant amount of support during this time. Because all these decisions were difficult ones, we believe that collaboration and joint problem solving helped us come to analytical, ethical, and professional decisions that took into account both the well-being of the patient and the difficult matter concerning the dog.

In dealing with discharging the couple, our team had to face two primary challenges. One was that Mrs. K could no longer take care of Mr. K because of her stroke. The other was their eviction from their apartment and loss of their belongings. Mrs. K continued on to rehab to regain the use of her limbs affected by the stroke. In addition to adapting to his new role as caregiver to his wife, Mr. K was striving to regain control over their lives and living arrangements. Joint physical assessments took place with the therapists and patients from both teams working to teach the patients how to adapt to their disabilities and responsibilities. The social workers met and spoke with each other almost daily to discuss housing issues and the search to find new housing. The unit administrator, social worker, nurse, physiotherapist, and occupational therapist consulted regularly to solve problems and address the challenging behaviors Mr. K demonstrated. He was extremely anxious, refused to be involved in the process of searching for new housing, and hoarded food items on the unit.

Our organization came together to help this displaced elderly couple. Our patients lost the belongings of a lifetime when their apartment of forty years was condemned as a public health hazard. All of us worked to restock and furnish their newfound home with donated household items. The kitchen staff, housekeepers, senior management, volunteers, staff who worked in allied health, spiritual care, IT, human resources, and occupational health all contributed items. A wheelchair technician used his own vehicle to move the items to the new apartment and helped to unpack and organize the couple's new home.

All of this was possible because we moved from a singular to collective and collaborative point of view that involved numerous departments in the organization as well as several local agencies and community services. We treated the patients both individually and as a couple. I have worked in many settings over the years—acute care, the community, long-term care—and in comparison with my varied experiences with interprofessional teams, this particular case epitomized the definition of "teamwork" and "collaboration," as the patients' successful discharge would not have been possible if each patient had been represented by a "team" operating on its own. The take-home message of this case is not that heroic action must be taken to save patients. What it does show is that teams that have established the infrastructure of collaboration can—when necessary—go extra miles in their effort to ensure that their patients are safe. When health care workers function in a system and culture in which they can rely on one another's specialized skills, they can better assess, treat, and assist people in complex situations such as that of Mr. and Mrs. K.

On January 13, 2012, Mr. and Mrs. K were successfully discharged back into the community to a new furnished apartment. Mrs. K had regained most of the use of her arm and leg. Mr. K successfully adapted to his new role as caregiver to his wife. Referrals were made to several community agencies to assist with follow up, case management, and in-home personal support. Both patients are managing well, and Mrs. K continues to visit our Outpatient Stroke Clinic for ongoing therapy.

· · ·

CHIARA CAMPITELLI-THOMPSON, MSW is a Social Worker who works with elderly patients in Geriatric Rehabilitation and Providence Healthcare in Toronto.

The "Nice" Patient Who Distrusts Our Best Advice

Nelli Fisher

In summer 2011, a labor and delivery team including myself (a perinatologist), two anesthesiologists (one of whom did the original consult and the other who was present during the delivery), an obstetrician who attended at the delivery, a nurse, and a midwife cared for a patient who posed a series of critical dilemmas. Our patient (we'll call her Joan) was a lovely thirty-three-year-old woman who was pregnant for the first time with twins. Always nice and polite, Joan, however, consistently refused our advice, which was that she deliver her babies in the hospital and not at home, as she wanted.

This was a serious problem because Joan was going through a high-risk pregnancy. She had a thyroid mass in her neck that would make intubation in a crisis very difficult. As the pregnancy evolved, first one of her twins—and then both—presented in the breech position—that is, the lower part of the baby's body was coming out first instead of the usual "head first" delivery. Both Joan's thyroid problem and that fact that her twins were breech made hers a high-risk pregnancy. She was a definite candidate for a Caesarean section and certainly needed to be delivered in the hospital.

On learning that there is a very high of risk of mortality—both for mother and babies—most people accept our advice on having a hospital delivery. When I, as the obstetrician who handles high-risk pregnancies prior to delivery, talked with Joan at our first clinic meeting, she refused to consider a C-section and insisted on continuing with her plan of having a natural birth at home with a midwife. In fact, at our first meeting, she told me she had only come to the clinic because she wanted to get her medical record so that she could take it to the midwife who would deliver her at home.

I listened to Joan outline her preparations for a home birth and politely but firmly told her that if she didn't agree to deliver in the hospital, both she and her twins could die. She would not budge on her decision but agreed to return to the clinic for prenatal care. Over the course of the next nine weeks, I continued to meet with her and to try to convince her to deliver in the hospital.

I recognized not only that this patient needed my best practices but also that I would have to work with a team. I thus asked the anesthesiologist, Dr. Oksana Bogatyryova, a warm and experienced physician and mother, to talk with Joan. When Oksana spoke with Joan, she explained that she understood her concerns and anxiety. She assured Joan that she would take care good of her in the hospital. She went on to explain why the mass in her neck could pose a problem if she needed general anesthesia, which could occur if the babies went into fetal distress. The safest approach, Oksana explained, would be to plan a C-section with regional anesthesia. Joan again refused. It was frustrating for both myself and Oksana. Why, we wondered, would a patient refuse to change her plans once she heard about the danger to herself and her babies?

We also informed the operating room nurse, Coleen Orilio, about the patient so that she could be prepared in case the patient came to the hospital after an unsuccessful attempt at a home birth. If Joan were to start delivering at home and there was cord prolapse or a drop in the babies' heartbeat or bleeding, or any other problems, this would be a real emergency. For example, a problem with the babies' heart rates would mean that the only option would be general anesthesia, which, in turn, would mean she would have to be immediately intubated. Because of the mass in her neck, this would be very difficult. So the labor and delivery team, including an OR nurse, needed to know about this.

In spite of our concern, Joan was adamant and committed to delivering at home. She believed that her home midwife was an expert in the delivery of twins. Again, I explained that no one who is expert at delivering twins could promise a safe delivery for twins in breech with a mother who had a serious thyroid mass. I repeated the facts: if anything went wrong, there would not be time to get to the hospital and deliver the twins safely. I also reiterated that not only were her babies at risk but she was too.

In our discussions, the patient would sometimes equivocate, saying she needed to talk with her boyfriend or her family. But she would never bring her boyfriend or any family member in to see us so we could explain the dangers to them. As the pregnancy advanced, we became increasingly concerned. I even began to have nightmares about the case. What if she carried out her wishes to deliver at home? What if something went wrong? What if everyone died? She did not seem to share any of our fears. Her strong beliefs didn't seem to be cultural, religious, or political in origin. It was her first child and, compared with giving birth in her own bed with a caring midwife, the hospital represented a sterile and invasive environment. Joan wanted an entirely natural childbirth—no IVs, no epidural, not even fetal monitoring to make sure the babies were safe.

As the perinatal attending, I spent a lot of time putting myself in the patient's shoes. I imagined how all the medical procedures and equipment in our hospital could be perceived as unwelcoming and disturbing to this woman whose life would soon change. I tried to make sure the patient came to her appointments, didn't have to wait, and had all the attention she needed. I discussed her situation with the head of labor and delivery, Dr. Sandra McCalla. Joan met with Dr. McCalla, who assured her that, should she agree to deliver in the hospital, we would have midwives available to be part of the team taking care of her. We told her that it was possible that the first baby could spontaneously turn into the head down position which meant that, even if the other twin was still in breech, she could deliver vaginally with the help of a midwife and an attending obstetrician. I made sure to have her meet the hospital midwife, Phyllis Lynn, the director of midwifery, so that she would feel more confidence in the team. I fully briefed the midwife, and we talked with the patient together. The midwife encouraged the hospital delivery. The patient listened to her politely but left the meeting without fully committing to a hospital delivery. Subsequently, the patient called Phyllis with questions. Finally, we gave the patient the names of doctors at Maimonides who were experienced in delivering twins vaginally. She didn't call them.

One day, at a clinic appointment, Joan was starting to have contractions and was 3 cm dilated. Her waters were still intact. I knew that once her waters broke, if the cord prolapsed this would severely compromise the blood supply to the babies and an emergency C-section would have to be done within minutes, which, because of the mass in her neck, could be a catastrophe. Alarmed, I said, "There is no more time to decide. I am driving you to the hospital. You know you can't have a safe vaginal delivery. Let's go."

When we arrived, the patient was greeted by the obstetrician, Dr. Stefan Novac, and the attending anesthesiologist, Dr. Kalpana Tyagaraj. At each step she continued to be nice but to delay the epidural and to refuse the IV. She didn't actually request that the hospital midwife be in the delivery room but had communicated with her over the phone. Finally, she began to demonstrate her trust in the team, and she allowed us to put in an IV and give her an epidural. Eventually she had a Cesarean section. Mother and babies were safe. The team could finally breathe a sigh of relief.

The next day, the midwife helped her with breastfeeding. She hugged the nurse and thanked the anesthesiologist and prepared to go home to her new life. She agreed to follow-up visits and didn't seem upset that she didn't get to have her home birth. In fact, when we had her first postpartum visit, she actually thanked and hugged me.

This good outcome would never have happened without this extraordinary team. We could have all given up, each one of us saying we gave her our best advice and that's all we could do. We could have tried to get a psychiatric consult to say she wasn't competent to make this decision. We could have lied to her and been paternalistic to make her comply. We could have handed her off to other team members. But we didn't. We suffered with her and for her. We tried to mobilize our humanity along with delivering expert medical care.

This experience and the good outcome has become part of institutional learning at Maimonides. During Schwartz rounds, a bimonthly forum where teams present their emotionally and socially challenging cases, we presented this one. This case was very compelling. Many people in the room understood from their own experience how hard it is to establish trust, to deal with someone who is "nice" but isn't moved by the team's concern. They also understood the challenge of dealing with one's own frustration when the patient doesn't change his or her behavior based on the severe risks he or she runs. What if there wasn't a safe alternative or a possible good outcome?

In the end, the team was relieved by the patient's acceptance of their recommendations, but the stress was at times insurmountable. The questions we all asked ourselves were: Would we invest like this again? What did we learn that could help us deal with future patients? Will we remain open to searching for answers and growing professionally? As one of the team members confided:

> I am still not very sure how best to provide safe care when the patient disagrees with us because of lack of trust—whether the origin for the mistrust is cultural, personal, religious, or some other cause. Reaching out sounds good, but many times options are limited because of time constraints. Then what? Should the providers be nice, polite, agree with the patient, and cross their fingers for a good outcome because of a miracle? Or should they use stronger approaches like obtaining mandates from the state or court. . . . I don't know what else. I still don't know the answer.

· · ·

NELLI FISHER, MD is a Maternal Fetal Medicine Attending and Director of Maimonides OB/GYN Simulation Program, Maimonides Medical Center, Brooklyn, New York.

Teamwork Is Part of Our Duty to Advocate

Jillian Chandler

I came in to start my day shift as a relatively novice nurse on the respiratory unit where I had worked only a few times as a float nurse. As I received the shift report from the night nurses I took note that one of the patients I was going to be looking after that day, an elderly woman with chronic lung disease, was requiring a lot of extra oxygen to help her breathe. "Don't worry," the night nurse told me, "the doctor is aware of the situation and saw the patient; she will be fine." When I entered the patient's room to do my initial assessment and take vital signs I noticed that the patient was anxious and was breathing very heavily and rapidly. Despite the supplemental oxygen that she was receiving through the plastic tubing inserted into her nose, she appeared to be in respiratory distress. The patient's daughter was also at the bedside and was distraught.

"What is going on?" she asked. "My mother was fine when I saw her yesterday."

While trying to stay calm and focused, I checked the patient's oxygen saturation. If the level is too low the patient can become "hypoxic," and the organs can start to die due to a lack of oxygen. In this case the patient's oxygen saturation was 80 percent, well below the 92 percent level we want to see. Still trying my best to remain calm, I placed a face mask on the patient and began to increase the concentration of oxygen delivered through the mask until her oxygen levels began to rise. Finally, her oxygen levels returned to normal, but she was requiring a very high concentration of supplemental oxygen, much higher than she did the day before. This was a significant concern. If her oxygen levels started to fall again, the next step would be to move her to the intensive care unit and place a tube down her airway to help her to breathe artificially. I did not think this was the ideal scenario for this elderly patient, and I could see that both she and her daughter were becoming increasingly anxious. I tried my best to reassure them, and then I left the room and headed to the nurses' station.

Because I was a float nurse and not a permanent staff member on that unit, I was unsure whom I should approach for help. I paged the resident who was looking after the patient, but she was busy elsewhere and said she would stop by later in the day if she had time. I knew the patient had to be looked after immediately, but the doctor was insistent and I began to doubt myself. Maybe the patient would be all right and I was just overreacting. After all, I had very little experience in this area, and the night nurse did not seem concerned. Still, I felt uneasy, so I sought out the charge nurse and explained the situation to her. To my relief, she accompanied me to the patient's room to take a look. Once she saw the patient, she knew, as expert nurses do, that this patient was in trouble. She knew the patient from previous shifts and recognized that this was not her "norm."

She immediately sprang into action to get the patient what was needed. "I will go page the respiratory therapist and the critical care outreach team," she said. "You keep the patient and her daughter calm." Within a few minutes the respiratory therapist (RT), a health care professional who specializes in caring for patients with respiratory issues, was at the bedside assessing the patient and taking blood samples. Moments later, the critical care outreach team (CCOT) nurse (an ICU-trained nurse on call who can assess a patient and determine if an ICU transfer is required) was also at the bedside.

After assessing the patient and reviewing her chart, lab results, and other relevant information, the RT, CCOT nurse, charge nurse, and I discussed what needed to happen next. Due to the chronic and degenerative nature of the patient's condition, things were not likely to improve, and we all agreed that discussions needed to take place with the patient and family about what level of care they wished to receive. In other words, the patient was likely to die in a matter of days or weeks if she did not receive a lung transplant (which she was not a candidate for) or get transferred to the intensive care unit and placed on a ventilator. Alternatively, the patient could opt to forgo any invasive treatments and receive palliative care, the goal of which is to relieve suffering and improve quality of life for patients in their final days or months. We also agreed that other team members would need to be involved in such discussions to ensure the patient and family were fully informed before making such an important decision.

I paged the resident who was caring for the patient to discuss the situation. She agreed that we needed to reassess the plan of care and came to speak with the patient and her family. The charge nurse also paged the advanced-practice nurse from the palliative care team, who came to offer her perspective to the discussion. Following the discussion, the patient and her family were understandably very emotional. The patient had decided not to undergo any more invasive procedures, and the family was dealing with the fact that their loved one was near death. The palliative care nurse and the resident explained the types of interventions we could offer in order to make the patient more comfortable.

When the rest of the team had left, I stood in the room with the family and the patient for a while, mostly in silence. Throughout the remainder of my shift I returned to the room frequently to ensure that the patient remained comfortable by administering medication to decrease her secretions and make it easier for her to breathe. I frequently assessed her respiratory status and pain level. At the end of the shift the patient and her family thanked me, and I felt I had made a difference in a very difficult time in their lives. I also learned a valuable lesson that day about the importance of teamwork and drawing on others for support. I learned that as a novice nurse there is a great deal I don't know but that there are many individuals within the interdisciplinary team who are willing to help out. I began to see that no single discipline has all the answers but that when we apply all our unique perspectives to a situation and work together we are able to provide exemplary patient care. I also understood that in order to access this interdisciplinary expertise I had to value my own judgment about a situation that made me uncomfortable. What I learned to do that day was act on those feelings in a way that helped to create the bedside team that got this particular patient what she needed to navigate her last days of life.

· · ·

JILLIAN CHANDLER, RN is a Patient Educator on an inpatient Psychiatry unit in Toronto. She is passionate about nursing and nursing issues and is also involved in the Registered Nurses Association of Ontario (RNAO). She was a fellow in the Collaborative Academic Practice Innovation and Research Fellowship Program at University Health Network.

A Second Chance

Illana Perlman

Monday is always the busiest day of the week for me. Nine years ago, I experienced a Monday that was no exception. As the social worker in the trauma unit of a large urban teaching hospital, I had been urgently paged to meet with the parents of two newly admitted trauma patients. The sisters, Sarah, twenty-two, and Lisa, twenty-four, had been in a motor vehicle collision when the car in which they were traveling was struck by another vehicle that had crossed the center line and collided with them head on. They had been airlifted to our trauma center, and their parents and younger brother arrived within a few hours in a state of disbelief and shock.

Sarah was intubated in the critical intensive care unit, having suffered a severe brain injury, a chest injury, and a lacerated liver. Her initial score on the Glasgow Coma Scale was 4. (The Glasgow Coma Scale is a neurological scale that aims to give an objective way of recording the conscious state of someone for initial and subsequent assessments. The total score is 15, so the lower the score, the more severe the brain injury.) Sarah was exhibiting decorticate posture, a sign of severe damage to the brain in which a person is stiff with bent arms, clenched fists, and legs held out straight. Lisa was in the step-down intensive care unit where patients are not on a ventilator or life support and there is a patient-to-nurse ratio of two to one rather than one to one. She had chest injuries and a spine fracture for which they applied a halo vest, an orthopedic device to immobilize the neck and head that is attached to the skull by pins. Sarah was certainly the more critical of the sisters, and for two weeks her brain continued to swell and her condition deteriorated. At one point, she had to undergo emergency neurosurgery, and the "guarded" prognosis was changed to a "poor" prognosis. Her pupils were fixed and dilated, and she had no gag reflex. I remember the meeting clearly; I sat with her parents and the intensive care physician as he told them that

Sarah had a less than 10 percent chance of survival. He suggested that they consider the withdrawal of life support and presented the issue as if the decision needed to be made quickly. I expected that they would reach that decision with some haste.

I met with the family two to three times per day, providing support to them throughout this critical time. We quickly developed a strong bond as is often the case at a time of crisis and vulnerability for our patients and families. In my social work role, I represent the one consistent staff person at a time of enormous anxiety and uncertainty in an overwhelming hospital complex that comprises multiple units and a myriad of constantly changing physicians and nurses. I was frequently the interface between these parents and the various team members, ensuring an awareness of key information and care plans.

The admission of a critically ill relative to an intensive care unit creates considerable anxiety and stress for family members. Medical and nursing care focuses primarily on maintaining the physiological stability of the patients, while social work focuses on meeting the emotional needs of the patient and family. The team also looks to the social worker for clarification of the wishes of the patient and family, as well as their informational needs. Understandably, it was very challenging for this family to attend to Lisa's recovery at a time of uncertainty about whether or not Sarah would survive. I informed the parents about the hospital's staff, procedures, and communication processes and assisted them with practical matters, such as accessing insurance benefits and legal aspects, discharge planning for Lisa, and linking them with resources that they needed to sustain them.

The hospital became their home, and for days they slept in the waiting room, keeping a vigil at Sarah's bedside. Their level of crisis was immeasurable as they experienced a rollercoaster of emotions with the fluctuations in her condition. Despite Sarah's decline, their faith was unwavering, and to know them was to know that they would not easily withdraw life support. Although her voice trembled, Sarah's mother's words were strong and resolute in responding to the physician during that pivotal meeting, and I can still hear them now: "I waited nine months for my daughter to be born; I shall not decide to end her life in an afternoon." That meeting triggered significant turmoil for this family, and it was in this context that I engaged one of the most significant interventions of my social work career.

I had walked into that meeting with the same approach that I had for most meetings in the critical intensive care unit: to be a support to the family, an extra pair of ears, so to speak, particularly to ensure their understanding of the information presented. I was not aware that the focus was going to be on the possibility of withdrawal of life support. I believed it was for the purpose of updating the family on Sarah's condition. As the meeting progressed, it became clear that the physician was requesting that the family make a decision regarding withdrawal of Sarah from life support. He explored the severity of the injury and the likely long-term impacts on her quality of life, presenting statistics in this area. He also shared a personal story from one of his own family members in a similar situation, which I believe was a reflection of his empathy.

A physician's role in leading end-of-life decision-making conferences for families in the intensive care unit is an extremely delicate one. The physician is working in a climate of pressure for access to limited beds (often referred to as "rationing") and balancing the delivery of information to families about the very sensitive issue of their child's condition. Studies have emphasized that strong communication skills are critical, particularly the ability to listen, to give families time to absorb the information, and to provide them with emotional support in the process. At times during the meeting I felt as if I were walking a tightrope between supporting the family in their state of immense shock at the choice with which they were being presented and ensuring that their perspective was being heard, while still working collaboratively with the physician who was pressing them to make this life-and-death decision.

In facilitating the close of the meeting, I summarized the parents' perspective and their evident need for more time. After the meeting, the physician took me aside and expressed his dissatisfaction at my "undermining" his meeting with the family. As we debriefed, I clarified that my role was one of support to families, irrespective of their decisions and that he was misinterpreting my joining with this family as working counterproductively to his perspective. I affirmed the family's position on withdrawal, which I had learned over the two weeks of getting to know them through numerous conversations, to help him understand that their approach prevented them from making any "quick" decisions, regardless of the information he had presented. This situation reinforces the importance of role clarification and mutual understanding and respect among health care team members as critical components of effective collaboration and teamwork in a hospital context.

Leaving that meeting, I experienced an uneasy realization that this family did not have sufficient medical information with which to make this grave decision, irrespective of the path that they would choose. While they had met with the intensive care physician and heard from him about their daughter's condition and limited potential for a quality of life, they had not spoken to the neurosurgeon and had not received details more specific to the brain injury and the prognosis. I knew that for the family to live with whatever decision they made, it would be essential for them to be able to look back and know that they had obtained all the necessary and relevant medical information and that they had weighed it all in order to reach the best possible decision.

I shared my concern with the family and set about advocating with the intensive care team to engage the neurosurgeon on the case to review the patient's condition. That afternoon, I contacted the neurosurgeon and set up a meeting with him and Sarah's parents. Within a couple of days, the neurosurgeon had reviewed Sarah's chart and test results and had given the parents his perspective on her prognosis. He also engaged a colleague neurosurgeon at the hospital to provide an independent consultation on this matter. I was present with the parents when they met with the neurosurgeon and received his information, which was in fact in direct opposition to that of the intensive care physician. In short, he stated his belief in the patient's potential for recovery and a quality life, however uncertain, and said that he did not support withdrawal of Sarah from life support at this time.

This was a whirlwind time for this family, within the raging storm through which they were already living. They clearly communicated to the intensive care team their intent to continue all care for their daughter and stayed with her day and night, moving into our hospital's hostel in order to be close at hand. Sarah underwent a tracheostomy and a feeding tube insertion and remained in intensive care for several more weeks. This was a particularly dark period for the family, following on the heels of that meeting with the intensive care physician. During this time, Sarah's mother shared with me her fear about what she knew she would need to do, out of respect for her daughter, if they had made the "wrong" decision and Sarah did not emerge from the coma. Sarah had been so intensely vibrant and vital with such a zest for life. They knew that she would not want to live in a persistent unresponsive state.

We waited and wondered, and Sarah remained unconscious for six weeks. It was a struggle for this family to cope, given that both parents were staying at the hospital, sleeping in our hostel, and taking turns at Sarah's bedside day and night. In between they tried to visit Sarah, but they felt torn because their major anxiety was related to Sarah's survival but, although Lisa was not critical, she certainly also needed family support.

Slowly, Sarah emerged from the coma and started to respond to voices. She began to move purposefully and to track her visitors. She started to engage with her family and with our therapists, first in gestures and then verbally. Our team was incredulous at her recovery, and the neurologist who had first assessed her to have a poor prognosis in the critical intensive care unit returned to reassess her on the trauma ward. He documented her recovery as "remarkable . . . she is alert with mild aphasia . . . good comprehension, fluency . . . good limb movement . . . walking . . . eating."

Miraculously, Sarah had beaten the odds. Two months after admission to the trauma unit, she was discharged from the hospital into the care of her family, where she continued to receive extensive and intensive community rehabilitation for several years. Her long-term injuries include being legally blind, suffering from constant vertigo, and not being able to taste or smell. As a testament to her strength and resiliency, she returned to school and is now a registered holistic nutritionist. She is also a motivational speaker, regularly presenting at our hospital's injury prevention program that targets high school students and is aimed at reducing risk-related trauma in youth. Both Sarah and her family acknowledge the "second chance" that she has been given in life.

Decision making about treatment continuation or withdrawal for patients with severe brain injury involves tough discussions about the benefits and the burdens, and about outcomes that are difficult to predict. While Sarah experienced a substantial recovery of cognitive and physical function, her outcome could also have been an early death or survival with extreme physical and cognitive disabilities. In these situations, although the outcome may always be in doubt, what should always be clear is the need for interprofessional discussion, such as that which I facilitated for Sarah's family. The concept of interprofessional education is developing as an integral component in the training of health care professionals throughout Canada; it emphasizes the importance of effective collaboration and teamwork for the efficiency and quality of health care delivery. In the hospital context, social workers are particularly well positioned to champion and facilitate teamwork and collaborative practice among members of the health care team, given their training, their close alliance with the patients and families, and their role and function in the Intensive Care unit and other units.

I have worked in the trauma unit for more than twenty years, and while many situations arise that speak to the importance of interprofessional communication and collaboration, the experience of Sarah and her parents is an exemplar for several reasons. First, it highlights the critical importance of ensuring that all families receive adequate medical information related to an injury and sufficient time in which to absorb this, particularly when difficult decision making is involved. Second, it emphasizes the importance of advocacy in working to support families during hospitalizations. Indeed, it is incumbent on every member of the health care team, irrespective of their role, to act on behalf of the patient and family, especially if one believes that there is a concern, such as supporting a family's need for more time or, if there is a gap in information, to facilitate their obtaining that information. Third, it emphasizes the importance of ongoing interprofessional communication among the members of the health care team to ensure mutual awareness, ongoing respect, and the understanding of the patient and family perspective. Respecting one another's professional perspective is a cornerstone of effective teamwork. It also minimizes the potential for tension through misunderstanding or misinterpretation of actions, as was the case when the physician considered me to be undermining his position. Hospitals and health sciences schools throughout North America are recognizing the need for and benefits of interprofessional practice, both in terms of enhancing patient care and more satisfaction among health care workers.

As a result of the experience with Sarah and her parents, the practices and processes for our communication and teamwork in the intensive care units have changed for the better.

· · ·

ILLANA PERLMAN, MSW is a clinical social worker in the Trauma Program at Sunnybrook Health Sciences Centre, Toronto. She has held this position for twenty-two years, specializing in crisis intervention and adjustment counseling with patients and families who are experiencing life-threatening injury. She is also an Adjunct Lecturer at the Factor-Inwentash Faculty of Social Work, University of Toronto, and is responsible for coordinating all facets of the social work student education program at Sunnybrook Health Sciences Centre.

Taking Care of Tom and Ethel

Heather M. Young

Discussions of teamwork and interprofessional practice in health care tend to focus on hospital work. Teamwork and interprofessional practice, however, are essential to good outcomes no matter what the setting, whether it be hospital, home, or in the kind of community-based long-term care organization where I have spent much of my career as a nurse and leader. Few stories can better illustrate why teamwork is so important in community-based care than the story of Tom and Ethel.

Tom and his wife Ethel lived in a large home in the mountains in the Pacific Northwest. Tom, who was eighty-six, was a retired humanities professor. Ethel, who was eighty-four, was involved in a variety of community causes. They had one son—Dan, a tax attorney in his midforties, who lived several hundred miles away. Dan, who had a stressful life of his own, was very concerned about Tom and Ethel and their ability to live independently.

Tom and Ethel had a rich and complex life and, to Dan, an utterly chaotic existence, which made him regard them with a combination of affection and exasperation. His parents didn't eat at specified mealtimes but when the fancy struck them. They were night owls who felt perfectly comfortable driving to the supermarket at 1 a.m. because there were fewer cars on the road and fewer shoppers in the market. Their house was cheerfully cluttered. Its rooms were always filled with music as well as lots of accumulated stuff. Every room spilled over with artifacts they'd collected, books they'd read or intended to read, rugs, blankets, and dozens of other objects, small and large. Dan thought of them as hoarders. To Tom and Ethel, the rooms in their house contained their life history as a couple.

Sadly, however, they navigated these rooms with increasing difficulty once Tom developed serious problems with his vision as well as increasingly severe Parkinson's disease, while Ethel had diabetes and was in the early stages of dementia. When Dan came to visit one Thanksgiving, he was very disturbed by what he found. The house in the woods, with its slippery decks, different levels, and relentless clutter seemed to him to hold a myriad of accidents waiting to happen. His mother seemed unable to pull together a Thanksgiving meal, and when he looked in the fridge, he found lots of ice cream and treats but not much nutritious food.

Dan, as I said, had never been comfortable with his parents' lifestyle, but now he was freaked out. Things that he could let go when they were in their fifties, sixties, or even seventies now seemed to be intolerable. His father seemed more frail, his mother more out of it. He didn't think that his parents' doctors were maintaining adequate surveillance and control. Something, he was convinced, had to change—and at once.

This is where I came in. At the time I met Dan, I was the chief operating officer of a retirement community near where Dan lived, where I designed a variety of programs. I was also the nurse practitioner running the community's clinic. Dan came to see us and outlined the problem and his expectations. He told me that his parents needed to come and move into our community. Then he delivered a list of their medical problems and what he wanted us to do about them. He wanted them to be in a safe environment. He wanted them to be supervised at all times. Their meds needed managing. They needed to eat right—that is, three squares, served at eight a.m., noon, and six p.m. He had a very clear concept of what was needed. To tune up mom and dad they needed to be in a very controlled world because they were, in his view, way out of control.

What was presented to me was, of course, a serious and compelling set of medical issues. It was also clear to me that this couple's rich life was now being refracted through the lens of Parkinson's, diabetes, and dementia. They and their needs were being totally medicalized.

I knew that there was much more to it than that. The issue wasn't how Dan or his proxies were going to manage his parents' meds. The issue was how these people were going to continue to live authentic lives. Throughout their marriage they had made choices that some would not consider to be the safest or most conforming. But those were their choices, and just because they now had grey hair and some significant disabilities, did that mean it was time for Dan and his proxies to completely take over?

I knew that when Dan moved them to us, which he soon did, our team would have a very interesting challenge. Our philosophy of community-based long-term care was clear to us. In a retirement community, a member's health and medical condition are a part of existence, but not all of it. Once Dan and Ethel came to our community, they would live here, take their meals here, and engage in social interaction here. Transportation, food, relationships, entertainment, exercise—all of that and much more would happen here and they would probably not be leaving—at least not until they died. Our job would be supporting, facilitating, providing or preventing, and brokering. Our goal would be to recognize that, as with so many couples who have lived together for decades, we were not dealing with a single patient but with a linked unit. As we soon discovered when they moved in, for example, Tom was the brains in the couple and Ethel was the brawn. When they had to do laundry, Ethel carried the basket down to the laundry room, put the clothes in the machine, and turned the dials—as Tom guided her. Tom would prompt Ethel to take her insulin and monitor her blood sugar. They were totally intertwined, and because of this the way to ensure that they were both optimally healthy was to help them continue to function together for as long as possible so they could, as they had always done, augment each other's strengths.

That was not, however, how their son viewed us, his parents, or the place where his parents had come to live. His view was that his parents needed to be controlled individually and that they had come to live in our community only for medical management. So the tensions were clear from that first meeting.

They only increased when Tom and Ethel finally arrived, along with their truck full of belongings and a massive old car they'd been driving for years. To put it mildly, there had not been a lot of sorting when they cleared out their 3,000-square-foot house to move into a one-bedroom 750-square-foot apartment that had only a small kitchenette. They arrived with more boxes than we had ever seen. Their apartment was filled with boxes from floor to ceiling. One of the first challenges was where to put things and how to get them to unpack, hang the pictures, and sort things out.

This was linked to the more fundamental challenge of helping them adjust to a place where meals were at certain times and medications delivered at certain times. We had fire codes, which meant dealing with clutter, extension cords, books, and their other things. There were all these new boundaries that they never had to deal with before. Plus, they had lived a very connected life. They had friends, they entertained, they were involved in a community, and here their only social contact was their son, who was busy and had his own family to deal with. So here they were in a place with all these rules and structures, none of which they had signed up for, negotiated over, or felt they had even chosen for themselves.

One of the first signs of the challenges to come occurred one night when a nursing assistant called me at midnight to tell me that when she went to check on Tom and Ethel, they and their car were nowhere to be found. We had worried about their car since their arrival. Tom was nearly blind, so Ethel, who was demented, drove while Tom navigated. Their driving during the day was worrisome to staff, but leaving in the middle of the night without telling anyone they were going was more so. We called the police, who finally located the couple in a nearby Safeway surfing the ice cream freezer and loading up a basket with pints and quarts. What was the problem, they wondered? They'd always gone shopping at night. Needless to say, when their son found out about their escapade and the fact that we had, in his view, allowed them to escape, he hit the roof. And to add insult to injury, why were we allowing his mother to have ice cream when she had diabetes? What kind of guardians were we?

What was, of course, going on here, in this incident and in their lives as a family, was that parents and child had very different visions of what should happen in the older couple's life as they began to decline. We were the intermediaries, and we had to balance their safety and their autonomy while sensitively dealing with their son's concerns. To do all this required not one person but a highly coordinated interprofessional team that included not only people we traditionally consider to be professionals—nurses, doctors, social workers, physical therapists—but nursing assistants, maintenance staff, receptionists, housekeepers, and others.

One of the first things we did to make sure they were safe was to help them unpack their boxes, sort through their belongings, and put things in a secure place. To do this we involved one of the maintenance staff—Mike. Working with Mike, we devised a workable strategy that would allow for the unpacking without invading Tom and Ethel's lives. Mike wouldn't simply knock on their door and announce, "Hi, I'm maintenance. I'm here to unpack your boxes and hang up your pictures. Let's get to it!"—something their son clearly preferred. Instead, he got to know Tom and Ethel as they walked around the facility. Then he would drop in to check on them and casually say, "Hey, why don't we hang up some of those paintings while I'm here." Because Mike was genuinely interested in the couple and very friendly, they accepted his help.

The same was true with the housekeepers. We knew that it was important for Tom and Ethel to accept their help. We also knew the housekeepers could make sure there were no dangerous cords to trip on or rugs to fall over and that they could check to make sure the couple had enough nutritious food in the fridge. Tom and Ethel, like many people, resisted having their sheets changed and their house cleaned.

So the housekeepers would come and help and then tell Ethel that they knew it was important to her to do the laundry herself, but hey, why not let us change the sheets and launder them—after all you're paying for it, why not take advantage. This was important to us not only to make sure the sheets were clean but also to ascertain whether Ethel had any problems with continence. Given this approach, Ethel agreed, and we were, later on, able to determine when she did develop such problems.

The housekeepers who earned Ethel's trust would also say things such as, "Ethel, you know there's an exercise class in twenty minutes. I'm going over there; do you want to come with me?" We knew a knock on the door telling Ethel it was time to get over to her exercise class and "I'm here to take you, let's go" would not have worked. But this approach that gently integrated help into the fabric of her life did.

Nursing assistants were critical in helping Tom and Ethel reconstruct a social life. We got Tom hooked in with a group of men with whom he would have coffee in the morning and discuss the news. I knew a nursing assistant who loved reading who asked Tom to go with her to the library where he could get audio tapes or large-print books while she got books for other residents. Ethel loved getting her nails painted. She was also physically active. Working with nursing assistants, we got her linked to an exercise class as well as connected her with a women's gathering in the afternoon.

Dealing with Tom's son became the job of a social worker. What we helped Dan to understand was that the couple were making conscious trade-offs. For example, Tom, who was very sharp in spite of his condition, explained that if he took his Parkinson's medication exactly as directed he would feel foggy. He would thus weigh his choices and titrate his dose. His calculus was, he explained, "If I fall every now and then that's okay with me. I would rather fall than feel totally out of it." Tom also titrated Ethel's doses of sugar. She was in her mid-eighties, after all, so why shouldn't she have some ice cream now and then?

To manage the tensions around autonomy and safety and our own liability—after all, state regulators could come in at any moment and say we were violating standards of care—we had to involve everyone. We had to deal with clinical issues with the couple's primary care provider, with the nurse practitioner on staff, with the specialist physician who was managing Tom's Parkinson's and Ethel's diabetes, with the dietitian who helped manage Ethel's diet, and with other staff and outsiders involved in their care.

In fact, dealing with the couple was so complex that early on we took their case to our ethics committee because almost as soon as they arrived, I could see that caring for them would only get more complicated and that there would be problems because of the conflicts over autonomy and safety and how rigidly you adhere to an institutional or medical schedule. I wanted to make sure we never lost sight of who they were. I knew that the best chance we had to get to know them was when they walked in the door, because I knew that although Ethel would experience a cognitive decline more quickly than her husband that he would as well. I wanted to make sure we understood their preferences and who they were as a couple before they got to the point where they couldn't express things as easily.

Here again, teamwork was critical and tremendously helpful. An attorney served on our ethics committee, and he quickly became a member of the care team. At each juncture of their care, he helped us understand our obligations as a facility as it pertained to licensing regulations as well as our duty to our clients to serve them in the way they chose and valued. One of the things he pointed out that was particularly helpful was that we had to make sure we were documenting well, so that any decisions that could be questioned were recorded and well communicated on the team.

Tom and Ethel lived with us for six years. Ethel and Tom lived together in the assisted living unit for three years, and then Ethel moved to the dementia unit. A year later, Tom moved into the skilled nursing facility because he was falling frequently and simply not interested in prevention. We tried to get him to wear a helmet, but he refused. We wanted to lower his bed and have a mat on the floor, and he refused. To the bitter end he was authentically himself. Yet this caused significant problems with the allocation of staff resources when they had to manage his injuries and take him to the hospital to get stitched up time and again.

Throughout their six years with us, teamwork allowed us to strike a good balance. Tom and Ethel were able to settle in and be themselves in this new environment despite significant life changes. Dan finally became part of the team once he gained trust in us and appreciated that caring for them wasn't as simple as he initially thought. But none of this would have been possible without an interprofessional team—not just one made up of traditional professions. Everyone on each shift took responsibility for supporting this couple to be themselves and to thrive as much as possible. From reception to housekeeping to the nursing staff, all were engaged in our vision of optimizing health in the broadest sense—to protect each person's authentic self.

Issues in retirement communities can be surprisingly complex. There is rarely a quick solution. In this case, it took about a year to problem solve and establish a solid plan of care with the endorsement of the couple, their son, and our staff. As a leader I had to prioritize. I had to sequence the issues and address the most urgent first. Various people on the team would say, "this is the most important thing; you have to deal with this right now," and you would have to look at the whole and at the trajectory to see a solution. It couldn't be solved all in one sitting. I am a big believer in creating balance among competing issues and allowing the tincture of time to operate so that the best solution develops more naturally and is not forced in a way that is hard to live with. It involves a commitment to a longer conversation that unfolds over multiple encounters and builds relationship as well as solutions. I cannot think of a more rewarding way to practice nursing with my interprofessional colleagues.

· · ·

HEATHER M. YOUNG, PhD, RN is Associate Vice Chancellor for Nursing, founding Dean of the Betty Irene Moore School of Nursing, and Professor of Internal Medicine at UC Davis. She's a nurse leader, educator, and scientist, and a nationally recognized expert in gerontological nursing and rural health care. Her career has spanned academia and roles in practice, leadership, and policy in community-based long-term care.

Hospital without Walls

Rebecca Quirk

The pediatric oncology nurses and physicians first met four-year-old Grace and her family when she was urgently admitted and then diagnosed with a malignant tumor in her abdomen. The family lived a simple life. They had animals—goats, chickens, and cats—and her father worked on their small farm and was upgrading their home in his spare time. Grace loved her animals. She had an infectious laugh and a way of peering at you through her thick, Coke bottle glasses. Her mother was about thirty-three weeks pregnant with the couple's second child. They had been anticipating a second natural birth at home with their midwife and young daughter present. The family had never been separated, and from the beginning of their time with us, their care presented a challenge. What could we do to support their wish for a simple birth and keep them from being separated any more than absolutely necessary? For a family with no outside resources, what could we do to meet their many, varied needs over what we knew would be an extended stay in the hospital for Grace?

The physicians, nurses, social worker, and others involved wholeheartedly embraced the concept of family-centered care. We not only needed to meet the physical, emotional, and medical needs of our four-year-old patient but also we needed to support her parents. In addition to helping to care for Grace, her mother needed to take care of herself as well as her unborn baby. Grace's father needed to quickly upgrade their home to be able to potentially bring home their increasingly technology-dependent, critically ill child, as well as a newborn—all while traveling back and forth between home and the hospital to be with his small family as much as possible.

The treatment team quickly realized that we would need more than our usual resources of pediatric oncology nurses, oncologists, and pediatric oncology social workers to meet their ever-evolving needs. Our team set up meetings with upper administration; staff in the nutrition department, including, dieticians, nutritionists, and even the people who deliver food trays; and, of course, labor and delivery/maternity nurses and an obstetrician as a precaution. The parents were invited to attend and were included in all final decision making.

Friends of the family donated and delivered food to help defer food costs. We got a small fridge for their room. The nutrition department was able to work out a plan to give extra food to the family at no cost to them. Working with their midwife, the family found a friend nearby who was willing to let Grace's mother deliver in their home just down the street from the hospital. The family had never been separated, and Grace's mother did not want to be separated from her any longer than necessary. She went to the friend's home for privacy for her checkups with the midwife. The mother and father also agreed to meet a local OB in case one would become necessary. We dubbed the experience "hospital without walls." Different departments and units worked together to help this critically ill child and her family.

Everyone needed to continually revise their plans as Grace's medical needs grew and became more complex. She required multiple surgeries and chemotherapy. The concerned treatment team grew to include more members and departments as we tried to accommodate her changing needs as well as anticipate and plan for contingencies.

Thinking outside the box, we constantly considered how we could mobilize our resources to keep this family together as much as possible. This meant that when the mother delivered her new baby, Grace would be cared for on the maternity floor rather than our pediatric oncology unit for the total extent of her mother's hospital stay. That, in turn, meant that Grace would receive any treatments that she was getting off our unit. The pediatric care team, made up of nurses, physicians, social workers, and other caretakers met with the nurse director of the maternity unit and experienced bedside nurses to see what we could do to accommodate the needs of a new postpartum mother and her baby as well as Grace on the maternity floor. When told the family's story, with their permission, the maternity postpartum staff were more than willing to try to accommodate the sick four year old on the postpartum unit.

As time grew nearer for Grace's mother to deliver, it became clear that Grace's cancer and chemotherapy schedules where not going to be cooperative. Grace was so sick and wrung out during therapy that we all dreaded that her mother would go into labor during one week-long therapy. Since delivering a baby is considered a relatively healthy process, Grace was definitely the higher risk, sicker patient. To coordinate the specialized chemotherapy plan, antiemetics, and to make sure Grace was safe, both oncology and maternity medical and nursing staff met at the administrative level. They decided that it was going to be much safer to have pediatrics somehow accommodate and care for the postpartum mother and newborn baby than to move Grace down to maternity.

We worked with the safety office and billing department. We didn't have a room in our oncology section that would accommodate two beds without violating fire codes. It was safer to keep them in the oncology section than to move them to one of the few double rooms in a different section of the floor. Officially and unofficially, we had to have a separate sleeping space for everyone involved. Working together during one of our team meetings with the pediatric care team, maternity staff, and the family, someone came up with an acceptable solution for Grace's mother—a well-padded recliner. With Grace's bed pushed up against the wall, a bassinet, a recliner, and the couch for Grace's father, we could meet fire codes and still accommodate the whole family. Grace's mother could lie down and/or sleep with Grace when they preferred and when all of her tubes and the comfort of both allowed.

I was caring for Grace on a Saturday evening shift when her mother went into labor while at Grace's bedside. For many reasons, the family had had to change their plans of delivering at the friend's house nearby. Grace's increasingly larger care team had brainstormed options with the family. The plan was worked out with the family and hospital administration to allow their midwife to assist in labor and be present at the birth in labor and delivery. In addition, Grace's mother consented to have an obstetrician involved. She labored in Grace's room, bathroom, hallways, and even the staircase outside the room. She tried, with the help of her midwife, to only go to L & D for delivery, but unfortunately, she ended up requiring a Cesarean section. A nurse and Grace's father brought Grace down to L & D four floors below to see her mom and meet her new baby brother. The parents had reluctantly agreed with the obstetrician and Grace's care team ahead of time that the new baby and mother would benefit medically by spending one night under the supervision of the maternity nurses who were better trained at assessing and intervening in the case of any OB emergencies.

When I returned on Monday morning, Grace's mother came to our floor, and I was handed the three care plans for my three patients in one room. Maternity nurses would come up at least once a shift to assess the mother and baby, but they were available for consult as needed; otherwise, they were our patients. I was responsible for providing the care that I was competent to provide—vital signs, physical care, emotional support, and meds as needed. Both units were responsible for paperwork, but maternity nurses were responsible for fundus checks and other activities with which I, as a pediatric nurse, was unfamiliar. Maternity nurses also provided teaching before and during the mother's "discharge." As an experienced pediatric nurse, I was very comfortable providing support for newborn care and breastfeeding, plus this was their second baby. The OB, the midwife, and the newborn hospitalist also did check-ins and assessments.

Grace had not been well enough to be discharged since her admission several weeks before. Her mother and new brother were "discharged" from their inpatient room to their temporary "home"—Grace's room—where they continued to live with Grace and her dad. Her mother still slept in the recliner or with Grace. The nutrition department continued to send trays to make sure her mother ate well so that she could heal and nourish her new baby. Grace's baby brother slept in his bassinet or with his parents—happily oblivious to the work that had gone into coordinating his birth and care.

About a month to six weeks after his birth, I realized that Grace's baby brother had not been to see his pediatrician yet. He was cared for immediately after birth by the hospitalist service, but his sister and, therefore, parents had not been home. After discussion with his mother, I got permission to call their pediatrician, who also had privileges at our hospital. On hearing the story of our "hospital without walls," the pediatrician agreed to stop and perform a check-up at the hospital on his way into work the next day as long as someone could obtain the necessary measurements to plot the baby's growth. I measured the baby's current weight, length, and head circumference and took a set of vital signs and faxed them to the office. The pediatrician came in the next morning on his way to work to meet and examine his new patient.

We held a hospital-wide lunch-and-learn gathering to review and discuss the coordination and care that went into taking care of Grace and her family. Individuals from different departments were invited to participate in a panel—to share their part and feelings about the "hospital without walls" experience. It was well attended by hospital staff and other departments—some who had been involved in the planning and carrying out of our "hospital without walls" and some who were curious about what the term meant. Other departments, outside of our pediatric and maternity floors and immediate care team, appreciated the experience of being involved in making a difference directly for a family. So many times, the care and work done by ancillary departments happens in the background and may go unnoticed and underappreciated unless there is a problem. Here, their contribution was recognized; they were invited and participated in the planning from the beginning. The lunch-and-learn was an opportunity to have their work openly acknowledged and for them to feel good about their contributions. The family was even invited. The parents attended and thanked the group. It was an emotional moment.

I wish their story had a happy ending. Grace and her family did make it home and in and out of the hospital a few more times before Grace closed her eyes for the last time. The family was extremely grateful for the extra care, time, and effort we put in to helping them live their lives as closely to their ideals as possible.

Providing care to this child and her family required an enormous amount of work, planning, and persistence. In pediatrics, we have always tried to do the kind of team building necessary to deliver patient and family-centered care on our unit. In this case, however, we needed to build a team that extended way beyond our unit. From this experience, we learned what it means when an entire hospital is involved in developing the kind of broad-based teamwork necessary to make care centered on the patient and family a reality throughout the institution.

. . .

REBECCA QUIRK, RN is a pediatric nurse, whose unit at the Barbara Bush Children's Hospital at Maine Medical Center cares for many oncology patients. At the time of this case, she was a Certified Pediatric Oncology Nurse. She has worked on her floor for twenty-six years and does a great deal of teaching with staff, families, and nursing students.

Alice Was Never Alone in Wonderland

Estella Tse

Alice in Wonderland had a simple fall, and it turned her world upside down but in a good way. Unfortunately for Mira, her simple fall in the back garden one evening in the spring did not result in a happy ending. She was elderly and lived alone but was functioning well in the community at the time of the accident. As a result of the significant brain injury she sustained when she fell and complications from a long history of smoking, she stayed in an acute care ward for eight months and was then transferred to a nursing home.

She had little family support and almost no visitors, but those of us who cared for her in the hospital learned that she had been a pioneer when she was living as a new immigrant to the country and raising three children on her own. Her common law partner of recent years spoke only limited English. Unfortunately, with his own health declining and walking becoming more difficult for him, he eventually stopped visiting a few months into her stay.

It was both hard and easy to work with Mira. We could have provided basic care that met the basic standards. Instead, we embarked on a journey that united a team of therapists, social workers, and nurses as well as support and administrative staff in the care of a very—albeit unintentionally—violent client. Initially, Mira was unresponsive, opening her eyes for short periods at a time but lying in a curled position most of the day. She was unable to communicate verbally because she had a tracheostomy and required oxygen and frequent suctioning. Ironically, our problems caring for her arose as the brain injury improved and she began to fight the staff. This would occur with bedside care, transfers to a chair, and during therapy sessions. Incident reports were filed about scratching, tube pulling, and kicking as the predominant themes. While many strategies helped to improve these behaviors, they persisted throughout her hospitalization and contributed to the difficulty in finding a suitable nursing home. In spite of this behavior, staff were persistent with Mira and struggled to provide a consistent quality of care without the use of restraints, as was the policy in our hospital.

In many respects she was not different from other elderly patients who have significant injuries. What was unusual was that, although she was so globally impaired, she exhibited moments of normality. For example, she could tie and untie knots in the ties of her hospital gown. In fact, she could meticulously unravel a whole line of knots created with IV tubing. In order to prevent unwanted activity with her gastrostomy tube, the staff started keeping her busy during the day with all manner of knots tied into bed sheets and then attached to her wheelchair. Certain staff even attained the title of knot master for the intricate kinesthetic bundles they created. Nursing and therapy staff noted an immediate calming effect on her from this seemingly purposeful task of untying knots. For significant periods each day, Mira no longer disrupted her feeding tube or removed her gown ties or fiddled with her seat belt. Eventually, this led to staff independently and thoughtfully sewing "busy aprons" and bringing in similar projects.

The physical and occupational therapists managed to see her together and achieved a reasonably safe mobility routine in spite of her continuing to hit and spit. They would distract Mira with soothing words and tones while trying to stay one step behind her. Full physical contact on both sides to help in a daily transfer to a wheelchair eventually translated into two circuits twice a day around the ward with assistant support staff. Mira's need to touch and grab meant that two staff always had to walk with her. In fact, all her care required this for safety reasons. In the midst of a busy acute trauma ward, individuals who were not even assigned to Mira's case voluntarily worked together to accomplish the day's tasks for her and offered encouragement when it was a particularly difficult shift.

One nurse in particular took a special interest in Mira's well-being, in part because of Mira's prolonged stay and her lack of family support. This nurse would bring in safe objects for Mira to manipulate, clothing that she would regularly launder, and even items to personalize her room. She accepted the challenge to be a primary care nurse and gladly showered Mira several times a week despite this being a particularly trying activity. I remember seeing a dark bruise on her arm from a pinch she got in one interaction.

There were countless meetings and ongoing informal group problem solving that led to strategies such as limiting unnecessary physical contact with Mira. Vitals and blood work were eliminated, as she was medically very stable. She was given a room near the nursing station so that many hands and eyes could minimize safety risks and provide the stimulation of friendly interactions. We checked equipment frequently for breakage, and cleaning staff monitored anything within her reach and sanitized things regularly due to her frequent spitting. Her need for oral stimulation prompted our speech-language pathologist to assess and reassess whether oral feeding could be a possibility despite repeated failures on bedside swallow exams.

I imagine that it must have seemed like the Mad Hatter's tea party from Mira's perspective, with staff presenting her with myriad colorful and creative objects, helping her to move freely and safely in a foreign environment, and addressing her with snippets of conversation that may not have had any meaning to her. In the process of trying to provide excellent care, we also learned that we could fail to safeguard someone's dignity. Well-meaning actions resulted in there being too much stimulation, and, as one social worker expressed, we were in danger of infantilizing Mira.

For example, there was no clinical reason to do her hair and put makeup on her if this increased her agitation and contributed to more negative outbursts. Simpler clothing could suffice for decency instead of fully coordinated outfits if it was a struggle to put them on her. Outrage about the lack of family involvement and our well-meaning overinvolvement needed to be tempered with the understanding that her children had legal power of attorney. Because of this we had repeated dialogue with the ethicist separately and with the family so that we could step back and appreciate choices that Mira would have made if she could have spoken for herself. With some tempering of her care plan and constant reflections that then led to adjustments in our thinking, we were able to achieve a balance that suited Mira. For most of her stay in our facility, Mira needed full care, yet once in a while near the end of her time with us, some embedded thinking pattern allowed her to escape from her wheelchair and start to do a normal task such as make her bed. In similar fashion, a day full of unintelligible grunts and grrs could be interrupted with an occasional "thank you."

In caring for Mira, we tried very hard to keep her needs—as well as we could ascertain them—at the center of our daily practice. This was not easy to do. But we could not have cushioned her fall down the rabbit hole without individuals who worked together as a cohesive team throughout what was a long, difficult, and ultimately deeply rewarding ordeal.

· · ·

EsteLLA TsE, OT is an occupational therapist for the Trauma, Emergency, and Critical Care Program at Sunnybrook Health Sciences Centre and has a cross appointment as Lecturer, Department of Occupational Science and Occupational Therapy, Faculty of Medicine, University of Toronto.

Part 7

BARRIERS TO TEAMWORK

Almost every health care institution, health professional school, and patient safety organization in the industrialized world has now made teamwork and interprofessional education, practice, and care a top priority. The World Health Organization's "Framework for Action on Interprofessional Education and Collaborative Practice" outlines the need for interprofessional work and the strategies and policies that will make it a reality.[1] The American College of Graduate Medical Education has announced that reforming health care depends on transforming the health professions. To participate in this transformation, the American College of Graduate Medical Education requires medical students to develop and demonstrate competence in interprofessional collaboration.[2] This is a new core competence for medical students.[3] The American Association of Colleges of Nursing and other health professional bodies have made similar commitments to interprofessional teaching and learning. Indeed, in 2012, six US health profession associations—representing allopathic and osteopathic medicine, nursing, pharmacy, dentistry, and public health—announced the creation of the Interprofessional Education Collaborative to further interprofessional education and care.[4]

The WHO document on interprofessional collaboration calls for a cultural shift in health care and argues that

> One of the benefits of implementing interprofessional education and collaborative practice is that these strategies change the way health workers interact with one another to deliver care. Both strategies are about people: the health leaders and policymakers who strive to ensure there are no barriers to implementing collaborative practice within

191

institutions; the health workers who provide services; the educators who provide the necessary training to health workers; and most importantly, the individuals and communities who rely on the service.

The WHO identifies the removal of barriers to collaboration as a key responsibility of health care leaders and policymakers. But what barriers are there to collaboration? Traditionally, these barriers have been too narrowly identified: Practitioners are educated and work in silos. Culture is the problem. Medical hierarchy. Poor communication. All of this is true. The stories in part 7 drill deeper to uncover how all of the above and more—particularly the organization of time and work—undermine some of the most well-intentioned efforts to practice collaboratively and form genuine teams. If those barriers are not removed, patients as well as those who work in health care will continue to suffer needlessly, and the real power of all the education, technology, and skill that health care has to muster will not be mobilized in the service of high-quality care.

The central theme in these stories is that health care hierarchies and concern with status and authority all too often trump patient care. Medical errors and injuries persist not because people don't care about patients or fail to intellectually appreciate the value of teamwork and team communication. One of the human factors that influences patient safety and people's ability to work on teams is our all-too-human propensity to go for the gold and to value as individuals what we value in our culture and society. If promotion depends on taking individual credit for the work that was probably done by a group, then it's not surprising that some people take that credit. If listening to a nurse (whom one has been taught to regard as an inferior) who warns about a patient safety issues means disregarding someone whom one has been taught to regard as a superior, then guess who may get ignored? If gaining status among one's medical peers means working with physicians not nurses, then work with physicians we will. If we are paid to work as individuals, then even for the most team minded of us, collaboration may be low on our list. And how can people work on a team if they have no time to learn teamwork skills and are constantly tired, frustrated, and irritable? In fact, one of the important messages of part 7 is that, in health care, many of the definitions of accomplishment and systems created to reward it actually penalize people for working on teams. What we have here is the proverbial good deed that never goes unpunished. That is neither a recipe for teamwork nor for good patient care. The stakes are so high that we must tear down these barriers.

Right Surgery, Wrong Patient? Wrong Surgery, Right Patient?

Frustrated Nurse

It's the first day of the new resident rotations in July in my well-known and well-respected teaching hospital. I'm charge nurse on our specialty floor, and the new R3 (third-year resident) assigned to the floor seeks me out to find out if we have a form for documenting a telephone consent for a procedure or surgery on a patient. The patient in question was not able to give the consent, and so the patient's husband needed to be called to provide it. The R3 and I checked the form and realized there was no "section i" for noting a consent that was taken over the phone. I then went to my patient care manager to ask about this, and she too was unaware of any place to document such a consent taken on the telephone and said she would follow up.

I went to report back to the R3 that neither I nor my manager was aware of a section in the form where a telephone consent could be recorded. The resident said he would manage to document the telephone consent on the current form. Because I was charge nurse and was not aware of any patient on my unit going to surgery (or having some other procedure) that might require a telephone consent, I looked over the form that he was filling out to see the patient's name. I noticed that the area where the patient identifier (with name stamp, medical record, and birth date) was supposed to be was blank.

"Which patient is this for?" I asked.

He said, "Don't worry about it; it's for a patient in the ICU, not on this floor."

Before I was even able to say anything, the new R3 slid the consent form over to a brand-new R2 (second-year resident) who was on this floor and service for the first time ever in his apprenticeship journey.

The R3 indicated that the R2 should sign the consent form as a witness to the consent—the one with no patient identifier on it.

I believe that part of my job is to mentor doctors-in-training, so I quickly spoke up and explained the perils of obtaining and witnessing a consent when there was no patient identified. This anonymous consent form—along with a signature that witnessed its completion—could travel up to the ICU, and the wrong patient's name could be inadvertently stamped on the form. A consent form meant for Mrs. Smith could be stamped with Mr. Jones's name. Or there could be two Mrs. Smiths, and instead of the consent form being used—as it was intended—for Lucy Smith, it might authorize Mary Smith to go to surgery and have a leg taken off.

Directing my comments to the second-year resident, I said, "Be very careful what you sign and what you say you witnessed when a form has no patient identifier on it." I used the opportunity to speak directly to the new resident. "This is how bad things happen and harm comes to patients." As this whole episode was unfolding, an attending physician was sitting at a computer nearby listening and saying nothing.

I left the room but was still worried. I knew the R3 still had to travel up to the ICU and get the right patient's identifier on the right consent form. I have no guarantee that that happened. In fact, his "Don't worry, I know who the right patient is" attitude was very disturbing. Not only could a patient be harmed, but future patients could be harmed because the R3 had bad patient-safety habits that he was also teaching the second-year resident. I don't know if my warning had an impact on the R2. What I do know is that, given the current hierarchy in the hospital, the R2 is socialized to listen to his mentor, the R3, not to the RN who just happens to come in and suggest that what his mentor is telling him is all wrong, against policy, and a threat to safe patient care. If he thinks that what I said makes sense, is he going to challenge the status quo and say, "Wait a minute, she's right"? In this case, he certainly didn't, nor did the R3 say, "Thanks for the reminder. You're right, this could cause a terrible mistake."

I hope my teaching had an impact. I have no idea if it did. In retrospect, I realize I didn't prevent any harm. What probably happened is that the resident went up to the ICU and labeled the consent form with the correct patient and nothing happened. If nothing happens this time, he thinks his risky behavior was just fine and will probably do it again. This is how deviance is normalized in our—and so many other—hospital settings.

But what is going to happen the next time? I realize that what I should have done to minimize the risk to this anonymous patient was to have said to both residents, "Wait a minute guys, this is a real patient-safety problem. Filling out and witnessing the consent for a specific surgery or procedure on a patient without the proper patient identifier is a recipe for a catastrophic error."

I could have gone on to explain that they were laying out the first layer of cheese that makes up James Reason's famous Swiss cheese model of error. Reason explains that in order for an accident to happen all the holes in the Swiss cheese must line up perfectly. In other words, serious accidents or harm to patients occur not just because of individual actions but system problems.

"What are we going to do about this?" I probably should have said, adding, "I need your assurance that you are both going to go up to the ICU together and go to the patient's bedside and look at his or her ID band and then, while you are at the bedside, look in the patient's chart and make sure that this patient is really the patient who needs this procedure. And then, while still at the bedside, you should label the consent forms. This whole process is backward. The consent should have been obtained after the form was correctly labeled and matched with the patient, not before. But if that's the way you did it, then what I am suggesting is the only way to safely deal with it."

I didn't do that. Why? Because in the world in which I work, saying this would be very difficult. First of all, I would probably get a lot of flack or pushback from the third-year resident. If I insisted on corrective action, I would need the energy and time to be persistent and make sure that it happened. If the resident were to blow me off and continue to proceed in an unsafe manner, I would have to then go up the chain of command, first to my manager, who might or might not be available and who, by the way, has no clear authority to deal with such a situation. I could then go to the chief resident, but I did not have the confidence that my concern would be taken seriously. So I did not pursue it.

When I left work, I was still worried about this deviation from procedure and concerned about my inaction. I thought about writing an e-mail alerting people to the problem, but I was not sure to whom I should send it. I could have contacted the chief of the department, the chief medical officer, Risk Management (who would be very concerned if they learned about this), the director of nursing, and so on. I could have spent the next hour writing a letter to the chief of the department and the chief medical officer making them aware of what others had done, my actions, and the risk I saw not only to the patient but to the new resident who—in the "see one, do one, teach one" model of medical pedagogy—was being tutored in unsafe practice. This was happening despite our knowledge that harm occurs on a global basis with over two hundred thousand patients dying every year because of medical errors and injuries. I didn't do any of this because I had no idea how this message would be received. Because of past experience, I didn't think it would be received well or that it would make any difference. I also didn't know that there was any mechanism for getting the lesson back out to the frontline staff and the new residents.

I didn't write any e-mails. About a week later, I had the opportunity to discuss this situation with the chief nursing officer and did write it up in an e-mail so that she could follow up with it at a monthly meeting with the chief residents. I hope this will have an impact. This incident illustrates something that happens with more than one set of residents deviating from safe practice related to accurate patient identification. I personally know of three other situations with other actors in which patient identification was either absent or not checked per policy, thus putting the patient at risk for error or injury.

In my discussions with nursing administrators and other nurses, the issue of our responsibility to immediately activate a hard stop when patients are at risk keeps coming up. In a culture of safety stopping the action and making someone aware they are about to make a potential error would be routine, expected, and received with gratitude and relief. In a culture of safety, I would have alerted the residents to their problem and they would have said, "Thanks for the reminder. You're absolutely right, we don't have clarity about which

patient we're consenting." The attending sitting at the nearby computer would have also chimed in and backed me up, commenting,
"Great catch!" We're a long way away from that, and I hope I'll have
the energy to keep trying.

· · ·

THE AUTHOR WISHES TO REMAIN ANONYMOUS.

Talking the Talk but Not (Always) Walking the Talk

Scott Reeves

Having spent almost all my twenty-year academic career—from research assistant, fellow, and scientist to professor and journal editor—focused largely on advancing our empirical and theoretical knowledge of interprofessional education (IPE) and interprofessional practice, I have witnessed a global expansion of interprofessional education and practice activities. Across the globe, interprofessionalism is a key movement in health care. It is therefore far more than the "flavor of the month"—a term used by some of its critics. Interprofessionalism aims to help address the fragmentation that has resulted from health professions whose education and practice has traditionally emphasized their separateness from one another. Interprofessionalism is a key mechanism to enhancing the collaboration and coordination of professionals to ensure they deliver effective, error-free care.

Many health care academics, and an increasing number in practice, now argue that IPE—in which professionals learn with, from, and about one another—will foster the competencies (attitudes, knowledge, skills, and behaviors) that enhance their ability to practice together and collaborate when delivering care. They also believe that this will ensure that patients will be provided with higher-quality, safer, and more effective care. IPE is also thought of as a tool that will help meet the changing needs of society—specifically it will help clinicians treat an aging population with complex chronic health needs. Finally, IPE is touted as a way to help address the rising costs of health care by reducing duplication through better interprofessional coordination.

IPE activities now span a variety of clinical contexts and involve a wide range of established professions (e.g., nursing, medicine), the emerging professions (e.g., physician assistants) as well as complementary professions, such as massage therapy. In the past twenty years we've seen an increasing evidence base from health care education and practice, which indicates that the use of IPE can be advantageous in enhancing the abilities needed for effective interprofessional practice.

This is all good stuff. And I have been delighted to be part of it. While health care academics are busy designing curricula that will create, enhance, and reinforce the interprofessional knowledge and skills necessary for future health care professionals to practice collaboratively, a central paradox remains largely unacknowledged and unaddressed. There has been almost no reflection given to the structures of academic collaboration and its role in knowledge production and dissemination.

A key element of importance to academics in their work is to occupy the principal investigator position on research grants or the lead/senior author on peer reviewed papers. Both positions are regarded as the most desirable and therefore most coveted, as they are counted as a direct demonstration of academic leadership. One therefore aims to secure these positions to advance one's career through the academy. As a result of this approach to undertaking academic activities, collaboration with others, in which roles and positions need to be shared with colleagues—one cannot always be in the prime position—is regarded almost as a zero-sum game, one in which there are "winners" (principal investigator or lead/senior author) and "losers" (any of other positions). Therefore, within this context, collaboration is not seen as a mutual and shared activity in which the processes are enjoyable and enriching, and products generated are of a higher quality owing to the input of different and diverse expertise. In other words, the sum is not viewed as greater than the individual parts

Consider, for example, how little real collaboration and how much of what I think of as "cutting out" occurs when people engage in writing a grant, submitting a paper, or preparing a paper, and colleagues exclude others in an effort to advance to a more prestigious academic spot. Or think of another phenomenon—what I call the "token effort"—that involves adding colleagues' names to grant submissions (sometimes without even asking them) to attempt to convey on paper a collaborative effort but where little or no attempt is taken to actually involve the person who was named. I have been in the field for many years and worked in several countries and have directly observed or experienced both of these phenomena myself or discussed this with colleagues. Both, of course, are frustrating, especially if you are on the receiving end of them. Both are also ironic—we are in a field whose aim is to promote and improve collaboration but that fails to do this because of these behaviors. Intriguingly, there seems to be a disconnect between what we practice and what we preach.

Part of this problem may be owing to a deep lack of self-reflexivity—a technique that one needs to learn to practice, and certainly to teach, interprofessional behaviors. This is a technique that can be taught and learned and that entails individuals reflecting on their social position or perspective in relation to others with whom they interact to develop an understanding of the possible influences involved when gathering and analyzing qualitative data—usually in the form of observations and interviews.

Perhaps more important is that, while we have been very rigorous about critiquing the fragmented evolution of health professional education and practice, we, as academics engaged in teaching and researching activities, have been less robust in challenging the very siloed structures of knowledge production, advancement, and status in health care academia. We have not engaged enough of a reflexive focus on the fundamental tension between the teachings of IPE and the behavior of its teachers who forge their careers in an academic world in which one's initial and subsequent scholarly challenges are dependent on the struggle to prove one's independent and original thinking, increase individual productivity, and demonstrate "leadership" with numerous scholarly activities. This also causes problems for health care students, who are trained to work under these structures. As a result, it continues to produce neophyte health care professionals who have seen how their professors operate—competing more than they collaborate. Although, in the academic setting, the impact of such behaviors is limited to possible career advancement, in the delivery of health care, its impact is far more significant, as failure to collaborate is quite literally a matter of life and death.

Attempts to transform the way academics in health care view collaboration and interprofessional teamwork need to focus on both the individual and the system. On an individual level, we need to develop the kind of reflectivity I have described. I try to do this personally and encourage it. When I am about to embark on a collaborative venture with new colleagues we have an explicit discussion about the anticipated processes and outcomes related to our collaborative work. While this helps reduce the chances of encountering collaborative problems, it doesn't necessarily eliminate them. Poor collaborative behaviors can still arise with colleagues during a project, but this approach helps ensure the collaboration starts on a secure footing. Then one needs to trust the verbal assurances while monitoring behaviors to see what actually happens over time.

More fundamentally, to make sure health care academics who teach future professionals do not subvert lessons in IPE we need to change the academic system to more effectively value collaborative activities (which do generate high-quality work). This will entail changing our academic criteria. For example, the notion of "original research" should perhaps be applied not only to the original research of one person but also to that which includes many. (Is there any research that is truly original and that isn't based on a foundation of research done—also, in part, at least, collaboratively—by others?) Our criteria could, in fact, shift to produce a "weighting" system for the different roles and contributions for the production of academic outputs. Of course, this paradox is longstanding and deeply embedded in the structure of all academia, not just health care, and so it will take dedicated efforts to introduce such changes. However difficult the mission, any movement to recognize and value interprofessional collaboration in the academy would surely help professionals move to truly interprofessional care.

· · ·

Scott Reeves, PhD is Professor in Interprofessional Research in the Faculty of Health, Social Care, and Education at Kingston University and St. George's, University of London, UK, and Editor-in-Chief of the *Journal of Interprofessional Care*.

No Good Deed

Darren Fiore

I am a pediatrician teaching at a large urban academic medical center where there has been quite a buzz in recent years about interprofessional education and collaboration. In fact, I even received a small grant from my institution to pursue a curriculum development project around the theme of interprofessional teamwork. At first glance, it would seem that our center is ahead of the curve when it comes to talking about interprofessional education. But what does it take to move beyond talk and actually motivate faculty to start teaching across professions?

In interprofessional education, we often talk about stretching outside of our "professional silos." This term refers to the fact that physicians are educated in their schools, nurses in their schools, and pharmacists in yet other schools. Often these schools are under the same physical roof, but they are independently administered and operated entities nonetheless. It can be challenging to branch out beyond these professional silos, in large part because of a gradual assimilation process that occurs to students during professional training. Doctors start to think like other doctors and pharmacists like other pharmacists. Interprofessional education aims to have members of professions learn with, from, and about one another. Let's focus specifically on some of the challenges in learning from one another.

Apart from traditional silos, there's an additional layer of culture that impedes opportunities for health care providers to learn from one another: the culture around professional and career advancement in academic medical centers. The old dogma in academia is "publish or perish," implying that faculty must be prolific researchers and writers to keep their jobs. This is how success is measured in traditional academic medicine. A faculty member writes X number of papers in Great Journal Y and presents her research at National Conference Z—this is the traditional formula for advancement. This paradigm gets a bit blurrier when it comes to educators in health professions. Is teaching valued as much as research? Is developing a course rewarded equally with developing a clinical trial? Is publishing in an education journal as important as publishing in a scientific journal? These are questions academic institutions, including my own, struggle with. If universities are grappling with these issues within their professional schools, imagine how complex it gets when trying to assign value to teaching across professional schools.

I recently attended a series of seminars for faculty at my university on interprofessional education. This was not a requirement; in fact my boss will probably never even know that I attended. I carved out the time to engage in this because the topic is interesting and important to me. I met a dedicated, experienced nurse practitioner who is using simulated patients to teach her nursing students. She was clearly hoping to meet folks from other professions who might be interested in helping teach her students. She said, "I talk to my students about interprofessional education during our simulation activities, but I feel like a hypocrite because I always end up having a nursing student pretend to play a doctor or pharmacist because it's just too hard to get an actual doctor or pharmacist to teach my class with me. Nobody has the time."

I sympathized with her plight. I am an educator with expertise in simulation; I do research in interprofessional team communication and, for goodness sake, I'm married to a nurse. I recognize and understand the importance of interprofessional education and collaboration as much as anyone. But time is a commodity in academic medicine. We have patients to care for, research to do, and medical students to teach. In order for me to take on a course teaching nursing students, even on a part-time basis, I would almost certainly have to give up something else. Would the university recognize or reward my time teaching in the School of Nursing? The answer to this is not very clear, at least to me. This means that individual faculty members are left to teach across professional boundaries at their leisure and at their discretion. This adds to the challenges of establishing sustainable interprofessional collaborative educational endeavors.

In sum, I would argue that when it comes to identifying barriers to learning from other professionals, the problem is complex. The old professional silos are part of the problem, but there is a deeper, murkier undercurrent that assigns a higher value to certain scholarly activities than to others in academic health professions education. "Doctors mostly teach student doctors" and "nurses mostly teach student nurses" seems to be the status quo. How to reward a nurse for teaching a doctor, a doctor for teaching a nurse, or a physical therapist for teaching a dentist hasn't been sorted out yet. Let's start to tackle that problem by publicly rewarding interprofessional educators, protecting their time to teach across professional boundaries, and recognizing such teaching activities as grounds for professional advancement in academic medical centers.

· · ·

DARREN FIORE, MD is Assistant Professor of Pediatrics at the University of California, San Francisco School of Medicine. Clinically, he practices as a pediatric hospitalist and is the Director of the Fellowship Training Program in Pediatric Hospital Medicine. His research interests are in medical education, with a particular focus on interprofessional teamwork and communication.

The Impact of Reimbursement on Interprofessional Care

Antonio E. Puente

Health care represents a little less than 20 percent of the gross domestic product of the United States. Of that 20 percent, about half goes to institutions such as hospitals and the other half to physicians and other health care providers. Individuals in the health care professions perform close to nine thousand different procedures; over one hundred different health specialties are involved in those nine thousand procedures. In essence, this results in about one million discrete possibilities that could be provided, hypothetically, to an individual receiving health care in this country. This number of permutations of health care possibilities is mind boggling, and the likelihood of efficiency, effectiveness, and measurable outcome decreases exponentially as the number of possibilities of health care procedures increases. Because physicians and other health care providers earn their livings by performing and receiving reimbursement for recognized procedures, the likelihood that clinicians will want to perform such procedures is high. Similarly, the likelihood that they will want to perform services that are not reimbursable is low.

These nine thousand different codes emerge out of a complex, scientifically based system of reviewing health care procedures, and they are compiled by the American Medical Association's Current Procedural Terminology (CPT) panel. The group comprises 120-plus advisers from the major health care groups in the United States (e.g., family physicians) who, in turn, provide their suggestions in a standardized, carefully developed empirical system to seventeen members of the panel. These seventeen individuals represent the industry (e.g., Blue Cross/Blue Shield), the government (e.g., Medicare/Centers for Medicare and Medicaid), and health care providers (e.g., the author). Established in 1966, primarily by surgeons, the group now covers the most qualified health care providers and services; their goal is to help determine which procedures are scientifically and commonly performed by health providers and, indirectly, how those procedures should generally be done. This system is used in the United States and Canada, as well as in an increasing number of other countries. In contrast, the valuing of a code (i.e., the actual reimbursement that the procedure or treatment receives) is determined by a group called the Relative Value Committee (of the American Medical Association). This is the other side of the CPT.

Of the close to nine thousand codes, most are focused on what health care practitioners do with, or do to, an individual patient. They are, to use the current jargon, "silo focused"; that is, the procedure is typically performed in a relatively isolated fashion. Though the codes imply and direct that the results of a particular procedure be documented, there are no clear guidelines that instruct the provider as to what she or he is to do with such findings and, typically, with a report. If a neurologist sends me a patient whom he or she believes to have dementia, and I evaluate that patient and begin to treat him or her, all that I am required to do is to send the referring physician a report saying that I saw the patient and found that he or she was indeed demented. That's it. There is currently no mechanism that encourages either me or the neurologist to communicate further about that patient. We are not required—nor are we paid except under highly limited circumstances—to communicate by telephone, e-mail, or in person, or to have a more extensive discussion about my findings and what she or he might want to do about them. More to the point, if we both decided such communication was essential, there would be a very, very limited way in which either of us could be reimbursed for the time we took to communicate to each other and to determine a mutual plan to deal with the patient and to engage in further followup. Though postservice work is captured in the valuing of such a service, the amount of work typically associated with such service is very limited and also is singular in nature. Collaboration between professionals is not incentivized and, typically, not performed.

The critical point here is that there is no financial incentive for one provider to communicate or to work together toward a common goal with another, not to mention with the many others who would be involved in caring for a patient who has multiple, complex problems—that is, most of the people we care for. For example, in the case of diabetes, there are no codes that encourage collaboration between an endocrinologist, podiatrist, psychologist, and primary care physician. In fact, in most cases, even access to such a patient's written records is still limited, though the advent of electronic health records should help alleviate this problem (assuming accessibility is available). This is because the decision about how the records are to be shared is left up to the patient to determine when filling out the HIPAA (release) forms at the beginning of a consult. When a patient comes into my office, it is she or he who determines the individuals with whom I am legally able to be in contact. This is the current situation, and it is hard to overstate how significantly this affects the goal of practicing interprofessionally. Educational and accrediting organizations, the Joint Commission, and others can make well-intentioned policy statements asserting that we should practice in an interprofessional manner, but if the financial incentives discourage this, health care professionals are not likely to encourage others professionals to join them in the common goal of a person's health. If diseases do not come in silent silos, why should health care?

The Affordable Care Act is, in theory, trying to change this reality. The new health care law encourages collaboration through several provisions such as electronic health records and health care homes. (In a health care home, a patient has a consistent team of heath care professionals who care for the patient in a collaborative fashion. The team is often led by a primary care provider.) Although the focus on interdisciplinary and coordinated care is central to ACA, the current CPT process is, unfortunately, not yet in congruence with the demands of coordinated care. Even if a practice creates a health care home for its patients, there is currently no clear financial mechanism to pay for collaborative care, because there have been no changes in the CPT codes that allow providers to bill and obtain reimbursement for integrative care. This is a serious concern, because so many of our patients come to us with multiple problems and are subsequently seeing multiple clinicians. Such communication is best achieved not only through the current standard of a printed or electronic medium (i.e., written charts and computerized records) but through other mechanisms, including telephone conversations and face-to-face meetings.

A paradigm shift must occur within health care and within the detailed mechanisms through which we pay for care if we are to relinquish the fifty-year focus on specialty and siloed care and to embrace a much larger vision that includes not only multiple medical specialties but all of those in the fields of licensed health care as well. Until then, CPT and ACA will be abbreviations for dreams not yet achieved. Whereas the reimbursement system is indeed evolving, it is shifting from the provision of services to paying for performance; collaboration is still not in the mix.

There are models all over the country of the delivery of coordinated care to patients. These are the interdisciplinary health care clinics that are funded by grants from foundations and private sources—not insurance companies—and that focus on truly integrated care rather than procedures. These, however, tend to be clinics that serve the indigent and presently uninsured. The Cape Fear Clinic, where I am among about 300 unpaid volunteers several times a month, is one of these models.

The Cape Fear Clinic is a multidisciplinary health care facility (including dental, medical, mental health, and pharmaceutical services) that serves southeastern North Carolina. In its two decades of existence, it has grown to serve almost 1,500 patients, with a budget of close to one million dollars. This is done with extensive grants from generous groups, such as the Cape Fear Memorial Foundation, the Reynolds Foundations, United Way, as well as numerous private donations, and the help of close to four hundred volunteers and a staff of one dozen. All providers share one electronic chart. Referrals for most procedures are done internally, mostly by forms, although sometimes by phone or even by walking the patient across the parking lot from one building to another.

Nobody "owns" the patient, and the patient is seen as an integral player in their own health care, from decision making to helping to contribute (as they can) to the clinic. The patient is not, therefore, categorized according to one particular problem; thus, there is no "mental health" patient, just Mr. "So-and-so" who has been vetted for income (i.e., 200% of poverty), residence (i.e., of one of the four counties served), and some form of identification indicating the county of residence. As necessary, when specialty procedures are required, that individual is referred to a specialist, who typically practices outside of the clinic and is willing to provide that service to the patient, along with documentation of the service to the clinic. The focus is on integrated, coordinated, collaborative care in order to increase efficiency, outcome, and satisfaction, while reducing costs as much as possible. At this point, for every one dollar the clinic receives, close to ten dollars worth of service is provided. Collaboration and interdisciplinary care are the solutions to the problems that silos have brought to health care.

While the Cape Fear Clinic is an excellent model for the future of collaborative care, I am concerned about how reimbursement will be obtained with the new ACA. Though in theory, the ideas espoused by the ACA are outstanding and innovative, the mechanisms to assure that revenue streams exist to support these ideas have yet to occur, at least within the current structure of the CPT system. Without appropriate systems of reimbursement, the future of the Cape Fear Clinic, and any other kind of interdisciplinary or interprofessional care, remains in doubt.

. . .

Antonio E. Puente, PhD received his doctorate from the University of Georgia. He has held several clinical and academic positions in the United States and abroad. He is currently Professor of Psychology at the University of North Carolina, Wilmington and maintains a practice in clinical neuropsychology.

The Time Trap

Suzanne Gordon

The other day, I had an amazing experience. I went to see my primary care provider, a physician named Jane Himmelvo, to discuss the pesky issue of my elevating blood pressure. As I age, it has gone from lower to higher—like 155/90 sometimes. The problem is, given what I know about health care and a terrible experience I had with a complication following surgery (one that my surgeon tried to blame on me and for which I received no apology, which would have been much appreciated), I have developed white coat hypertension. So whenever anyone takes my blood pressure in a health care facility, zoom, it goes way up. Jane and I have been trying to figure out how to get an accurate BP reading, and so I have been doing the readings at home.

So I was in Jane's office to report on the data I had collected. We sat and discussed it for a few minutes and noted that my regimen of aerobic exercise, lowered salt intake, meditation, and dealcoholized red wine was actually working, and we decided—and I use the word "we" deliberately here—that I would keep up the regimen for three to six months to see whether it would continue working over the long term.

With the problem addressed—at least temporarily—in about ten minutes, I was about to jump up and leave, knowing that ten to fifteen minutes is all you usually get with your PCP these days. But then Jane started asking some further questions. They were not: "How's your stress level?" or "Let's check that cholesterol one more time." She asked me how I found living in the Bay Area after having moved from Boston two years ago. When I told her I loved it, she asked about my kids. I asked about hers. We began to segue into our different ethnic backgrounds and religions. (I'm an eastern European lapsed Jew; she's a Vietnamese sort-of Buddhist.) We talked about prejudice, films. I kept peeking at the clock. I had exceeded my fifteen-minute limit ten minutes ago. Shouldn't I leave? But no, we kept chatting, getting to know each other. After forty-five minutes, our time to-gether seemed to naturally end, and I left feeling flabbergasted. Was she really a PCP? Was this really a doctor's visit?

Of course, she is, and it was. This particular physician has ar-ranged her practice so that she can actually spend time with patients. There's never more than one person in the waiting room at a time (rather than four or five). She never seems rushed or stressed or star-ing at her watch. And she talks with her face to you rather than with her back toward you and eyes glued to the computer screen as she hurriedly types in notes so she can get you out and the next patient—who's probably been waiting for an hour, because four patients have been booked for the same fifteen-minute slot—in. She also does house calls, which creates a fascinating dynamic in which the patient has a whole lot more control in his or her own home than in the doc-tor's office.

This is all done very deliberately. This particular doctor charges a $275 fee per couple per year (a kind of concierge fee) so that she can maintain a solo practice, actually get to know her patients, and have time to build trust. She also probably takes a cut in income and has to deal with the hassles she and her small staff experience. But she explained to my husband and me, when we had a meet-and-greet when we moved to the Bay Area and were searching for a new physi-cian, that she had begun to feel like an automaton in the group prac-tices that are the norm today. She wanted to do things differently, and she does.

Having been socialized in the new medical model of throughput, I found this all very strange for a while—as if somehow I'd landed on the wrong planet, even though it felt like a really good mistake.

I write about this because one of the things that is missing in dis-cussions of teamwork and patient safety is time. Physicians, nurses, pharmacists, and pretty much everyone who works in health care at any level today are working too long and too hard. They are taking care of too many patients, listening to too many histories, auscultat-ing too many lungs, charting the rhythms of too many hearts. When I began writing about health care almost thirty years ago, the average primary care doctor had a patient panel of maybe 800. Now it's up to 2,500, maybe even 3,000. At a major teaching hospital, which shall go nameless, some PCPs work from early in the morning till late into the night. Some actually sleep in their offices. This is not in India but California. In North America, resident hours have been reduced—a smidgen—but doctors who have finished their apprenticeship training have no restrictions on how long they can work, how much they should rest, and how many patients they can see, operate on, assess, and so on.

Years ago, in teaching hospitals, attendings and nurses used to be the safety net. Now, in all hospitals, everyone is stressed and overworked. Nurses, except in California and in some states in Australia, have no limits on the number of patients they can care for. As resident hours are reduced—somewhat—nurses' hours have escalated. While there are restrictions on how many hours truck drivers can drive their trucks or pilots and flight attendants work in their aircraft, there are none on how many hours a nurse can work. (Although most now work twelve-hour days, they actually are in the hospital for at least thirteen and a half.)[5] In most states there are no restrictions on mandatory overtime, and in none are there restrictions on voluntary overtime. Patients can thus be the sixteenth person a nurse is taking care of during his or her fourteen-hour day, and he or she can legally work that many hours on any number of consecutive days.

One of the reasons studies conducted years ago documented that nurse practitioners provided as good, if not better, care than physicians in routine cases was because they spent more time with patients.[6] That is no longer true today, as NP PCPs are pushed to be as "productive" as MD PCPs. And whether they are NPs, RNs, PCPs, MDs, PAs, PTs or any other combination of multiple letters in the alphabet, higher workloads mean more interruptions; and more interruptions, we are learning, mean more errors, since the brain actually doesn't multitask well. When forced to do so, it just does one task less well than the other task that it is supposed to be doing simultaneously.

The kind of stress people experience with these kinds of workloads is, we know, a significant barrier to teamwork. Stress makes people irritable, if not angry, frustrated, and possibly even abusive. Fatigue also has a serious impact on teamwork because it does the same. When people are constantly interrupted, they can become frustrated, particularly with the supposed team member—or patient—who is responsible for the interruption. Combine fatigue, stress, and something we are just learning about, hunger—guess what, the body needs food to fuel itself, just like a car needs gas, and when it doesn't get it, people become a little testy—and you have a proverbial perfect storm for poor relationships and poor communication, not to mention mistakes and potentially catastrophic failures.

Yet despite what we are learning about how the human brain actually works, health care shows little inclination to reduce workloads, work hours, workplace interruptions, or work stress. In 2013, I attended a conference on the patient experience in which physicians discussed their efforts to teach one another to be more empathic. The aim was to increase patient satisfaction scores and thus hospital reimbursement. The hospital in question was putting its physicians through empathy training. What it was not doing was changing their workload or work hours. Indeed, the physician presenting at the lecture emphatically stated that reducing productivity demands was off-limits and that nothing was going to change in that regard.

How precisely do you manufacture empathy if you are exhausted, have just moved from the thirty-fourth patient to the thirty-fifth, have not eaten for seven or eight hours (the body needs fuel more often than that or, silly thing, it begins to think it's starving), and are being constantly interrupted?

In its report on remedying the epidemic of medical errors and injuries, *Crossing the Quality Chasm*, the Institute of Medicine recommends that physicians spend time explaining how to take each and every medication they prescribe (or that has been prescribed) to their patients. But how, precisely, are they supposed to take a history, do an exam, be empathic, and go over the patient's perhaps ten to fifteen (or more) medications in a ten- or fifteen-minute visit? The report also insists that "the product of health care is not visits or 'encounters,' but healing relationships that allow patients to obtain the trustworthy information and support they need. . . . A patient with a question represents an opportunity, not a burden."[7] Really? In this environment?

In this environment, learning the skills of teamwork is also extremely difficult. Everyone involved in the pedagogy of patient safety and in trying to implement serious patient-safety initiatives—such as teamwork training—eventually confronts the issue of time. It appears in this form. There is no time in the curriculum for this or that. There is no time to teach this or that in the hospital. There is no time . . . (fill in the blank).

In 2013, I got a call from a nurse educator at a hospital who wanted to use the play I coauthored, *Bedside Manners*, in her educational efforts. The play is about the problems of teamwork and communication among health care professionals and other staff. These problems, she told me, were rife in her hospital. They were causing a lot of demoralization and were even linked to serious medical errors. But how, she wanted to know, could she adapt the play to the thirty-minute sessions she was allotted on the floors.

"Thirty minutes?" I asked incredulously. "Thirty-minute segments that occur over a period of weeks?" I queried.

"No, I get thirty minutes with a group. That's it. I don't get to come back," she replied. "That's life in an acute care hospital," she stated matter-of-factly.

I can usually be quite creative. But in this case I was stumped. I wanted to be helpful. But there was no way to make this work. None at all. In fact, were it not so tragic, the idea that you could possibly deal with complex problems and change well-established behaviors and attitudes in a one-shot thirty-minute session would have been almost laughable.

In health care everything seems to be up for grabs. We seem to be changing everything all the time. We are not, however, even broaching some of the fundamental obstacles to teamwork and safe patient care. The human brain can only cope with so much, even under the best of circumstances. And in health care people are usually confronted with the worst. They are dealing with patients who are sick, usually very, very sick, and thus frightened, anxious, grieving, sad beyond words, and sometimes angry, frustrated, and abusive. Working in health care is not like working at Macy's or the Cheesecake Factory or even Toyota. People come to health care providers and workers not because they want to but because they have to. Not because they want what is on offer but because it may be their last resort. They may not do what they are told, because to do so may involve something very unpleasant. Even with enough time, enough sleep, enough food, no interruptions, perfect knowledge, teamwork training and communication skills—and even rational reimbursement and reward policies—working with the sick is difficult. Without any of this, we have to ask ourselves, is teamwork and safe patient care a mission impossible?

Part 8

TAKING TEAMWORK INSTITUTION- AND SYSTEM-WIDE

Good teamwork, as we have seen in the majority of essays in this book, provides predictability and, thus, standard ways of delivering care. Creating good teamwork, psychological safety, putting the patient on the team and at its center, coaching, and removing barriers to teamwork can begin on individual hospital units or in individual facilities. To be sustainable and fulfill its promise, however, teamwork must be taught and normalized throughout entire systems. Similarly, when new things are learned during change initiatives, they must be shared throughout the health care system.

A 2013 *Health Affairs* article highlights how some health care institutions, such as Virginia Mason Medical Center in Seattle and Intermountain Healthcare in Salt Lake City, have done this very thing and achieved remarkable results not only in patient outcomes but also in cost reductions and improved efficiency.[1] Team-based approaches and shared decision making were some of the core principles allowing transformational ideas to succeed.

All of the stories in part 8 illustrate how institutions have tried to engage in the kind of broad transformation that creates systems that encourage people to work in teams by providing them with the skills necessary to do so. These narratives also highlight the power of "positive deviance" that Michael Gardam wrote about in part 4.[2] When leaders abandon top-down approaches and work to mobilize and unleash the imagination and creativity of the people closest to the patient—wherever that patient may be—amazing things that were hitherto considered impossible can happen. They can not only happen once but they can happen over and over again if team and institutional leaders remember that change (and genuine teamwork) doesn't just happen because a bunch of smart, well-intentioned folks get together and watch a PowerPoint presentation.

Throughout the world, health care systems, individual institutions, and those who work in them seem to be constantly asked to adjust to shifting institutional imperatives, job descriptions, staffing models, reimbursement structures, and professional and occupational definitions. Initiatives designed at the top are often imposed on those at the bottom, and even the traditional captains of the health care ship—physicians—now complain that they are no more than deck hands. When you add this to the complexity of patient care and the lack of stable relationships among caregivers, it is clear why it is critically important to incorporate the lessons from high-reliability, or high-risk, environments that have accrued over the last three decades.[3] The kind of institutional change described in part 8 makes those who now feel like they are merely the objects of change into the subjects who are leading the transformation, even if they have traditionally been invisible like the VA housekeepers described here by Rajiv Jain.[4]

In stories told by the caregivers, they themselves identify critical problems and develop tools and practices that use standardized communication and practices to improve teamwork and safety culture in a more predictable process. Top-down planning is eschewed in favor of including the perspectives and involvement of unusual suspects from housekeepers to patient transporters.[5] This captures the wisdom of those closest to the work and often to the patient. What is so impressive about these narratives is that many of them are taking place in large, complex systems or in radically different cultures. This teaches us that someone who has learned how to work on a team and honor other people's views can do so whether in Rwanda or the US health care system as the nurse Jessica Early discovered.

Addressing improvement in this way is far more likely to be successful and to result in measurable benefit and sustainable change than are top-down initiatives. Most important, the stories in part 8 debunk the myth that is all too prevalent in health care: that all that is needed to change established behavior is to expose people to new ideas on a one-shot basis. This deeply embedded belief in medicine nearly always fails to work.

Just as a jazz quartet learning new material demands persistence, practice, and repetition, so too teaching new behaviors in health care cannot happen without repetition, rehearsal, and constant coaching. Imagine what beautiful music (patient care) could be made if we simply practiced what we preached and if "co" really became cool.

Making the Handoff Safe in Labor and Delivery

Michael Block

As it is in many areas of the hospital, team-based care is a necessity in the fast-paced environment of a Labor and Delivery unit. Physicians and nurses are often confronted with unpredictable situations in which they have to interact well in order to manage patient care. One such interaction, which is universal in hospitals, is the patient "handoff" when physicians or nurses transfer care.

If handoffs are not well and carefully managed, untoward consequences for patients and staff often are the result. It is well documented that patients suffer harm when there is poor turnover between staff. Poor handoffs in Labor and Delivery units are linked to birth injuries. It is for these reasons that numerous national and international health care organizations and professional societies advocate the standardization of handoff practices.

The positive association between teamwork and patient safety is well documented in the patient safety literature. However, all too often, this literature tells us what to do but not how to do it. It doesn't give much guidance about how to deal with barriers facing the front lines such as constrained resources, professional hierarchies, and differing organizational priorities that may obscure the goals of having a team. The current approach to issues in L & D is often reactive and lacks objectivity—that is, structure, goal direction, and inclusivity of all stakeholders, especially frontline clinicians, is overlooked.

In our hospital—one that delivers over six thousand babies a year—we faced the challenge of improving handoffs and teamwork. For us, the opportunity to craft a handoff tool that would help meet the challenges of shift changes emerged after we had distributed the Safety Attitudes Questionnaire (SAQ) on our unit. This anonymous, simple questionnaire, which was developed by Bryan Sexton, Eric Thomas, and Bob Helmreich, measures local, unit-level norms through the lens of all frontline providers.[6] It asks staff about their perceptions of norms such as teamwork, safety, job satisfaction, and burnout. In a major breakthrough for teamwork on our unit, physicians and nurses got together in the same room to discuss the results of the surveys and identified areas where action could lead to significant improvement. When reviewing what the survey revealed about handoffs, they found that our unit scored poorly. It was clear that something needed to be done.

We knew we wanted to avoid two problems that can inhibit change. One is the problem of initiatives that are developed off-site and do not include frontline staff in their design, implementation, and evaluation. Instead of relying solely on recommendations developed off-site by people without knowledge of local work habits, we wanted to develop solutions that were grassroots and came from the bottom up rather than the top down. This, in turn, led to the second challenge. To create practical solutions we had to bring people together. Everyone's opinion mattered, and everyone contributed to the work.

To do this, however, was quite tricky. That's because when discussing unit problems there is a tendency to focus on one group of professionals or to single out individuals rather than focusing on system issues. In hospitals and in health care overall, for example, it's all too common to attribute errors to the individual providers' actions rather than re-evaluating the systems in which they are required to work. Statistically, medical errors originate from a lack of failsafe mechanisms in the systems within which caregivers work; that is, the systems lack inherent safeguards against human error. Clinicians are then blamed for these system problems rather than helped to change the systems. They are thus reluctant or afraid to engage in discussions about system problems for fear that they will be unfairly targeted. Or they may feel that nothing will ever change, and they give up trying to change anything. Because of the retaliatory reactions in hospitals, the possibility of learning (i.e., listening) from problems is often stifled. Clinicians tend not to report "near misses"—dangerous incidents that happened but didn't lead to visible harm. For all of these reasons, clinicians are often frustrated that initiatives may not produce real change, which, in their experience, means that the same problems will continue to resurface.

In L & D we knew that any initiative that involved handoffs would inevitably involve nurses because they spend the most time with patients and interface with physicians of every specialty. This meant that we had to include everyone involved with patient care on L & D together at the same table. The way we did it was to create an inter-disciplinary group that included nurses from each shift as well as obstetricians, neonatologists, and anesthesiologists. The use of the Safety Attitude Questionnaire helped avoid the finger-pointing problem by drawing attention to how everyone interacts in a system. It does so by the way the questions are phrased. The SAQ doesn't ask personally directed questions using language such as "you," "I," or "we" or questions that ask for a "yes or "no" answer. Rather, it elicits norms by asking participants to rate their level of agreement on a 1 to 5 Likert scale (strongly disagree to strongly agree) to statements such as "Information is communicated well at shift change" or "Physicians and nurses work as a well-coordinated team." This created a forum for conducting objective discussions that led to collaborative planning and action. It also helped us remain focused on our goal and attracted attention and support from unit leadership and hospital administration.

After looking at the data, we began brainstorming. In these sessions, everyone agreed that there were a lot of root causes to our problem. We asked the physicians, "What information from nurses is deficient when they are communicating with you?" We asked the nurses, "What's missing during your handoff from your peers?" We knew, for example, that when nurses exchanged information there was variation in conversational style. Handoff reports lacked structure because there was no standard format to follow. They were often done from memory or from jotted notes on scraps of paper or napkins. There was often uncertainty about clinical issues because these of this. Transfer of responsibility was not consistent because the transfer process from one nurse to another was neither defined nor visible. Sometimes care was turned over without a formal report, or sometimes a report was given but the information was not always accurate or up-to-date.

What emerged during our discussions of local practices was an agreement to turn our in-depth knowledge about nurses' work processes into our solution—to innovate. We deliberately rejected the suggestion that we create yet another electronic tool. When this possibility was raised, nurses said, "No, No!" They wanted a tool like a card that would encourage face-to-face encounters where they could see the expression on someone's face and have the opportunity to ask and answer questions. They also needed easy at-a-glance access to important information for carrying out patient care, which a computer screen could not offer them.

Since we knew that nurses were accustomed to writing things on those scraps of paper, the nurses in the working group suggested that we turn these scraps of paper into an SBAR (Situation-Background-Assessment-Recommendation) tool and pass it along when turning over care. The minute they suggested this idea light bulbs went off in people's heads. It was unlikely that this idea could have come from an outside consultant or other safety expert. People might have resisted it as we moved forward. Instead of feeling "They're making us do this," staff felt "Wow, what a great idea; we need and want to do this!" They also wanted to see the scores from the SAQ go up. They owned this project. We called it the "tangible handoff card."

Over a period of a year, we worked together to create a standardized, patient-specific, two-sided pocket card that would fold up and could be inserted into the pocket of nurses' scrubs. The card emphasized two components of the handoff—standardized communication and role clarity—including definitive transfer of professional responsibility. The tool could be utilized at critical transitions in patient care aside from routine shift changes. Examples include: (1) a patient nearing delivery, (2) a patient receiving an epidural, and (3) a patient going off to the operating room for a Cesarean section.

The tool we created together guides nurses through structured verbal reporting and acknowledging transfer of care and is updated throughout the shift. The front of the card formats information into a fixed SBAR 14 layout. General information, such as patient identification, location, admission indication, physician-contact information, and blood type, is incorporated into the "situation" header. Space to the right is used for noting reminders, concerns, and alerts. On the card's reverse side, categories of workflow-related elements (laboratory results such as blood type and screen, induction agents, antibiotics, tocolytics, infusions such as oxytocin and magnesium sulfate, and consent forms) are formatted with check boxes to draw attention to pending issues relayed at care transfer. The tool also includes final trigger questions (e.g., Did you address safety concerns? Did you conduct the handoff face-to-face? Did you notify the charge nurse about the handoff?) before handoff completion. Written endorsements (handoff time and participants' initials) and card transfer from one nurse to the next complete the transition of care.

To ensure that handoff reports between nurses address the total care for the patient, we integrated information priorities pertaining to the practitioners of the core disciplines in L & D (nurses, obstetricians, anesthesiologists, and neonatologists) into the content of the tool. For example, maternal and fetal status during labor (contraction pattern, fetal heart-rate tracing, and cervical dilation) relate to L & D nurses and obstetricians; patient comorbidities and pain assessment pertain to anesthesiologists; and gestational age, antenatal ultrasound pathology, and the presence of meconium are important for neonatologists.

Use of the tool begins at patient admission to L & D and concludes with patient transfer off the unit. A patient identification label is first applied. At the nurse's discretion, entries in pencil (to allow for changes) are placed as the care routine evolves. Typically, this coincides with patient admission, change in status, an intervention, or at handoff. Within-shift ("intrashift" or "cross-coverage") handoffs are verified with the L & D charge nurse. Following a verbal face-to-face report in a distraction-free location, each nurse initials the card. The time and type of handoff ("shift change" [S.C.] or "cross coverage" [C.C.]) are noted. The nurse assuming care for the patient keeps the card in a scrub pocket as a token of responsibility.

We spent the first three months of our work together developing the tool and testing it. We tested it on the night shift to see what worked and what didn't. Then we spent the next nine months evaluating it. Although we did not measure specific clinical outcomes, we did create and validate an instrument called the Coordination of Handoff Effectiveness Questionnaire to measure the quality of the handoffs. CHEQ results showed improved perceptions of handoff quality. It also showed increased levels of teamwork, increased levels of job satisfaction, and reduced feelings of burnout among L & D nurses. The cards are now used routinely for patient handoffs. Together, ten of the nurses and physicians who worked on this initiative wrote an article about it for the Joint Commission's *Journal on Quality and Patient Safety*.[7] We did this because we know we have a successful model that can be replicated by others facing similar challenges.

Because our initiative focused on a nursing process in a traditionally siloed setting, physicians could have absented themselves from the collaborative process, arguing, "What does this have to do with us?" Nurses could also have isolated themselves, taking a similarly siloed stance that physicians had nothing to do with a nursing handoff. In trying to create better communication between nurses and physicians, however, we discovered that almost every barrier to communication seemed to originate in a handoff—either because of unclear communication or ambiguous roles. It was thus critical for those at both the giving and receiving end of a nursing communication to be involved in improving the process. Our work together has not only created a replicable model that will enhance patient safety, it has also helped bridge team relations on the unit.

What the SAQ did was to hold up a mirror that reflected not individual experience but how the norms and expectations of the unit led individuals to interact as a group. We expanded the knowledge we gained from that exercise to innovate. Through that process, we united to form a cohesive team that now mobilizes to engage in teamwork around other patient care issues. Rather than just talking about teamwork, we began to create the infrastructure for teamwork so that people got into a communicating mode. This grassroots effort took a lot of time and patience, but it has helped us move toward a sustainable practice that is, in an era of electronic documentation, greatly valued and indispensible.

• • •

MICHAEL BLOCK, MD is an Attending Anesthesiologist and Director of Obstetric Anesthesiology at Hackensack University Medical Center (HUMC), Hackensack, New Jersey. He is a TeamSTEPPS Master Trainer, a member of the Quality and Safety Committee of the Board of Governors at HUMC, and a member of the Patient Safety Committee of the Society of Obstetric Anesthesia and Perinatology (SOAP). He was the lead author for the Tangible Handoff Project, an interdisciplinary program designed to measure and improve the quality of patient handoffs in Labor and Delivery.

Not the Usual Suspects

Rajiv Jain

Teamwork in health care is a complex and interesting phenomenon. When the words "team" and "teamwork" are mentioned, most clinicians think of team members either as people from their own discipline or from other traditional health professions such as nursing or social work. It is not uncommon for physicians to think they're doing a good job including people on the "team" if the medicine doc talks to the surgeon or if the surgeon talks to the cardiologist or pulmonologist.

Today, people intellectually understand that nurses and other clinicians need to be included on the team. Yet, nurses often complain that they are still too often excluded from physician rounds and decision making about patients they share. If physicians include social workers, nutritionists or dieticians, or physical or occupational therapists in their planning and decision making many of them feel: "We have covered social aspects, nutritional aspects, the physical aspects. We have a really good team. We are really good at team work!"

What this sometime inclusion of what I call "the usual suspects" leaves out are the "unusual suspects." These are people who are almost always overlooked because they are considered to be apart from the usual health care ladder. In many instances, their input may be crucial. This is particularly true when you're dealing with a difficult issue such as prevention of infections. To effectively prevent hospital infections, we must have a much broader concept of "team" than just its traditional clinical members.

At the Veterans Health Administration, we began expanding our definition of the team when we began to work on culture change in the context of preventing infection associated with health care. What we quickly began to understand was that we needed to include housekeepers, dietician aides, and nursing assistants who help to transport patients in wheelchairs or gurneys.

Why was this so important?

Consider just one example of efforts to prevent infections from the hospital "superbug" methicillin-resistant *Staphylococcus aureus* (MRSA). When we launched our effort to prevent MRSA infections at the VA Pittsburgh, we began by looking at the literature about patients who are admitted to the hospital who are not colonized by MRSA but who pick up this organism in the hospital. How does that happen?

You need only look at a hospital room to learn how. The opportunities for infection include the handlebars around the patient's bed, the table (which is equipped with drawers or sometimes mirrors) that slides over it, or the telephone. This is precisely where the housekeeper comes in. Housekeepers are the ones who clean what we call "environmental surfaces."

We did tests on patient rooms and found out that the housekeepers who were cleaning the room were not catching all of these areas. If a patient who had been in the room was MRSA positive, and the patient now in the room was MRSA negative, these trivial-looking surfaces were likely to contribute to colonization in the uncolonized patient.

The next steps were clear. If we succeeded in getting doctors and nurses and other health care workers to clean their hands as they should but housekeepers neglected to thoroughly disinfect the environmental surfaces, patients would get sicker. Housekeepers had to be included on the health care teams or our efforts to prevent MRSA would be in vain.

Instead of holding a meeting where we—the experts—laid down the law to the housekeepers, we held focus groups to share some information about how infections are spread and to solicit the input of housekeeping and other staff in the prevention of infections. An infection-control nurse visited various departments and asked simple questions such as: What do you know about MRSA? What do you do to prevent patients under your care from getting MRSA? What are the barriers that keep you from doing it 100 percent of the time? Do you know of anyone who has figured out strategies to overcome these challenges? If so, how? Do you have any ideas about new strategies? What would it take to implement them on this unit? Who is willing to take the next steps?

The approach known as Positive Deviance—finding a person who is not doing a problematic behavior and having others learn from his or her example—guided these queries. The concrete answers and broader responses to these questions drove the initiative.

One example of housekeeper involvement occurred during the early stages of the implementation of the prevention program. One of the housekeepers came to us and told us that we didn't have good protocols for cleaning the room after a patient who has a MRSA infection had been discharged. He pointed to the two types of cleaning protocols in the hospital. There is routine cleaning, which is done for a patient who has no resistant organisms and includes cleaning the floor and the bed, washing down the bed, and cleaning the counters. The other kind of cleaning is known as "terminal cleaning" and is used when patients have resistant organism. When they leave, housekeepers take extra time and wash down the curtain around the bed, clean inside drawers of tables, clean the phone in the room and all the things those patients use on a day-to-day basis. This is the only way to make sure everything is cleaned and disinfected properly.

This housekeeper told us that we didn't have a standardized protocol for terminal cleaning. The infection-control nurse and physician shared with this housekeeper's supervisor and other housekeepers the scientific and clinical evidence about what kind of agents they needed to use for appropriate disinfecting and how long they needed to use them. They discussed the right chemicals and concentrations. The steps came together, and then the group, with the housekeepers included, wrote procedures for terminal disinfection. The infection-control nurse and physician acted as consultants to help the housekeeping staff but not to dictate to them. This led to greater ownership. Housekeepers felt they had a critical role to play in protecting the life and welfare of patients. They wrote the procedures, they took—and continue to take—pride in making sure patients are safe. Here was the process in a nutshell: A housekeeper says there's a problem. He or she is taken seriously. The team involves other housekeepers. And they write the protocols and drive their implementation.

Once we looked at this issue, the housekeepers helped us to develop a protocol that was accepted by all housekeepers in one hospital. Then we moved out to the other 152 hospitals in the VA system. Housekeepers talked to their colleagues in other VA hospitals. We appointed a national group with involvement of the chief of Environmental Management Services. Then a national procedure was developed for terminal cleaning.

Housekeepers who had been involved in the Pittsburgh group were part of the national team writing procedures for the entire Veterans Health Administration. It was never "Thank you very much; now the experts will take over." When these protocols were introduced into the other 152 hospitals, the Pittsburgh staff, including housekeepers, was involved on a national level. But this was only part of the story.

DIETETIC AIDES

In most hospitals, large carts with heating elements and food trays move from one unit to the other as patients are fed. Dietetic aides (DAs) bring food to patients. Here again, environmental surfaces play a role in the possible spread of a superbug like MRSA. Imagine once more the table that goes over the bed. Before our intervention, the standard procedure was that the dietetic aide leaves the tray in a patient's room on the table and then goes from there to the next room. As part of this process, if the DAs don't wash their hands and don't gown and glove when they go into the room of a patient with MRSA, then they touch the table and become carriers of this organism. We repeated the same procedure we used with housekeepers with the DAs and came up with protocols that are now used throughout the system.

TRANSPORTATION STAFF

Finally, we had to consider the role of those who transport patients in the prevention of the spread of an infection such as MRSA. Because of HIPPA rules and other privacy regulations one can't tell the transport aide that a particular person has a MRSA infection. Yet, you have to communicate this information so that people take precautions when they transport a patient who is MRSA positive. The procedure we developed through the same process we used with housekeepers and

DAs was to send a gown and glove in the lap of a patient along with his or her chart. This communicates that the patient has some infection and that, to take care of this patient, one has to utilize standard infection-control precautions. It becomes a privacy-correct way of taking care of such patients and those they might infect.

The transport person will thus carry the gown and gloves so the receiving side (lab, X-ray) will know that they also have to take precautions by donning the gown and gloves. The role of the transport staff is thus to make sure that the person on the receiving side understands that the patient could contaminate others and that the gurney or wheelchair has to be cleaned when the patient is back on their originating unit. Because these protocols were developed by transport staff, they felt that they had ownership in them.

RECREATION THERAPISTS

The final step in breaking the chain of infection occurred when a recreation therapist came to us. Patients will go to their clinic to do activities to keep them engaged. Some patients may be MRSA positive. So this means that once they leave the recreation therapy area, tables and chairs and other items the patient touched would need to be cleaned. When the recreational therapist became aware of the program to prevent hospital-wide MRSA infection, she realized that she needed to develop a procedure for cleaning tables and chairs before a new group came in and after the new group left. Rather than keep this insight to herself, she came and talked to us about it and developed such a procedure.

Whether it is in one institution or many, culture change like this can only happen when infection prevention is everyone's business. This will only happen when we truly invite staff members—all of them, not just the usual suspects—to participate in this from the beginning. We did this in many ways. We shared information so that information about the problem was widely known. But we didn't stop there. We enlisted the people at the front lines as leaders—not champions or ambassadors who'd been chosen to promote the ideas of the "experts." They were the experts. We used focus groups—not newsletters or PowerPoint presentations—to disseminate information, and we solicited input from everyone. Physicians and nurses served as consultants, not dictators. We did this at one hospital, and when we had a successful model we didn't impose it on the other 152 hospitals— we repeated the process nationally. All of our ideas were shared through learning sessions and conference calls throughout 152 hospitals. Nationally, the infection rate in these hospitals was reduced by 65 percent.

This effort has not only reduced lethal infections, it has also created the infrastructure of genuine teamwork in our hospital system. We now have teams that include everyone—both the unusual as well as the usual suspects.

• • •

RAJIV JAIN, MD is Chief Officer, Patient Care Services, Veterans Health Administration and was the Director of the VHA MRSA Prevention Initiative.

The Art of Rounding

Lisa Fidyk

Ten years ago, I began my career as a neurotrauma nurse at the Hospital of the University of Pennsylvania. I quickly grew to love the hustle and bustle of the critical care arena. The staff worked well as a team, helping one another with the physical demands of caring for critically ill patients, offering clinical advice, and easing the high-stress environment with light humor at times. We called our unit the Fish Bowl because it was square in shape with glass rooms along the perimeter, and we could see into each room with ease. This worked to our advantage because we could witness when a patient's status changed or when a fellow nurse needed help.

I found the 2:1 patient-to-nurse ratio to be appealing because I was able to channel my energy when taking care of my two patients and could cultivate my critical thinking and reasoning skills. I appreciated the complexity of the patient population, the coordination of care provided, and ultimately the rush of saving lives. In the neurotrauma surgical intensive care unit nurses were heavily involved in the decision-making process of patient care, and thankfully we had good rapport with our physicians. I believe this was because neurosurgical residents did not rotate every several months as traditional surgical residents do; we were able to develop long-standing relationships with each resident.

I can remember long nights where the neurosurgical resident and I would be at the bedside caring for a critically ill patient. The resident would be placing a ventriculostomy as I tended to the patient's vital signs and prepared medications. We would converse about the next steps, which included packing up the patient to take to a computed tomography (CT) scan and maybe even neuroradiology. We were like a ship gliding through the halls, a passage we had taken a hundred times before. As the night would wrap up the resident and I would part for our separate ways. He or she would get ready to sign off, and I would finish my early morning tasks of drawing labs and freshening up my patients for the day shift.

As the new day arose, the physicians would proceed to round on each patient. Interestingly enough, this is where the collaboration ended. It was not uncommon for the physicians to read through the patients' charts, poke their heads into each and every room, perform a quick neurological exam and make assumptions as to how each patient did overnight without ever involving the nurses. It is not uncommon for a nurse to find on a neurological exam that a patient has experienced subtle changes in his or her condition—whether in their state of arousal, ability to move extremities, or to follow commands; I often wondered what important information the physicians missed by not checking with the nurses. In fact, I can remember having a list of things I needed to discuss with the physician only to get asked to save my questions or concerns for a later time.

Over time, the communication between physician and nurse became more complex as the physician hourly requirements changed. As residents were allowed to work only eighty hours a week, this decreased their time on the unit and increased the number of provider handoffs for those covering the patients. Around this time, we also introduced the role of the nurse practitioner. Having a nurse practitioner on the unit was a wonderful thing; however, there was confusion as to what needed to be addressed to the physician and what needed to be addressed to and by the nurse practitioner. Pertinent information was being missed, or nurses would inform both the NP and physician, which would result in double order placements or assessments by both providers. Our interaction with the physician or nurse practitioner resulted in role-accountability confusion. Also, our approach was reactionary in that nurses would bring forth a checklist of orders we needed from the physician or NP instead of having an open dialogue about the care of our patients. Our senior nurse leaders and lead physicians on the unit recognized the need for change that would increase standardization. After meetings with the neurocritical care team and nursing it was decided to have more structured rounding.

Nurses would present their patients during rounds. Yes, that is right! Nurses, not the medical student or resident who had to devote half their shift to the most critically ill patients or assist in the operating room. Because of their workload the physicians-in-training would run to the nurses' station right before 6 a.m. to quickly collect data from each patient's chart before the start of rounds. It would be the nurse who had cared for this patient for what might be several days and who knew the family and the intricate details of the patient's stay. It was the nurse who documented vital signs and made a neurological exam at least every hour, who bathed the patient and visually assessed every inch of his or her skin while conversing with the patient and noticing a slight change in speech or a new hand tremor.

Our staff developed a rounding tool to help guide the nurses in providing the patient information in a structured manner. In the morning, the attending would coordinate with the charge nurse the order in which the rounding would occur. At that point, the charge nurse would inform the nurses as to who would be starting rounds. Rounds would typically start around 9 a.m., which provided time for the nurses to receive report from the night shift nurses and assess both their patients and complete the rounding tool. Information on the tool included past medical history, allergies, medication list, events of the past twenty-four hours, assessment, lab values, fluid intake/output totals, and plan of care. Having nurses lead the conversation provided an opportunity for nurses to give an overview of their patients' status, raise any concerns, assess the plan of care, and develop daily goals with the team of physicians and nurse practitioners. It was a learning opportunity for nurses as now they were involved with the teaching that the attending physician provided. In addition, the residents and nurse practitioners now had more time to devote to patient care.

With any culture change there were obstacles to be faced. Nurses had to change their work flow to assure they would be prepared to discuss their patients even if unexpected events occurred prior to the start of rounds. Recognizing this as a challenge, the unit began to utilize a buddy system in which a fellow nurse would look after one patient as his or her partner presented on the other. In addition, the charge nurse would assess the situation and change the order of rounds if need be, as well as completing any remaining nursing tasks. In so doing, the neurocritical care team also grew to be more accommodating when unexpected events occurred. Another obstacle was the intimidation factor that nurses felt when presenting the patient data in front of a group of physicians who typically wanted concise information delivered in a certain fashion. To increase confidence and change the way in which data would be presented, the physicians and nurses worked as a team to modify the rounding tool to fit the needs of everyone. Consensus was made as to what pertinent data needed to be included and the order in which it should be presented. Through this process, the neurocritical care team of attending physicians, residents, fellows, NPs, and staff nurses developed a true partnership. Ultimately, it was a move in the right direction to ensure better collaboration among team members and to improve the safety and quality of patient care.

In time, the unit-based respiratory therapist, pharmacist, nutritionist, and charge nurse began to take an active role in rounds as well. This interdisciplinary approach allowed for improved coordination of care among the many disciplines and provided a clear picture as to what the patient priorities were for that day. As a nurse who embraced this change, I found myself having a clearer picture of the plan for my patients. I no longer had to call the physician or NP multiple times about an array of issues because all my concerns or questions were addressed during rounds. I also learned a great deal from the attending (and other specialists) as they would provide technical details of a disease process or the rationale for placing a certain monitoring device or staring a new medication. It not only allowed me to provide better care to my patient but it also contributed to greater personal and professional satisfaction.

I no longer work in the NT-SICU as I moved on to pursue a career in academia. However, I often revisit the unit where I started my career and have witnessed the rounding that occurs today. I'm pleasantly surprised to now see patients and families involved in rounds. The days where the patient's door was closed when the plan of care was discussed are gone. Doors are open, family members at times stand beside the health care providers, and open dialogue occurs in front of the patient. This model demonstrates that transforming relationships among professions as well as with the patient is possible.

With effort we can move from a model of disciplines working in silos with little information sharing to one in which communication, interdisciplinary collaboration, and family involvement are the norm. All it takes is a will and a lot of teamwork.

· · ·

LISA FIDYK, RN is Associate Program Director, Health Leadership and Nursing and Healthcare Administration Program at the University of Pennsylvania School of Nursing. She is also a Professional Development Specialist at the Hospital of the University of Pennsylvania.

Getting Everyone on Board

Francis A. Rosinia

Physicians have been taught that they are the captains of the health care ship, the leaders of the health care team. Sadly, however, few of us physicians are trained in how to lead a team or function as members of a team. As an anesthesiologist for the past twenty-five years and as chairman of the Department of Anesthesiology at Tulane Medical Center, I began to understand the dimensions of this problem two years ago when I was named chief quality officer at the Tulane Medical Center. As I examined the statistics on quality, both nationally and at an institutional level, it became quite clear to me that in our institution, as in any large hospital, enhancing patient safety meant tackling the fundamental issue that exists for any quality or patient safety initiative. That fundamental issue is, of course, culture change.

To make patients safer and to enhance quality, we have to act and think differently. In the area of quality and safety, acting and behaving differently requires not only physician buy-in but also physician leadership. Yet, when we tried to initiate safety and quality initiatives, we found that the default position of many physicians was that the hospital is responsible for everything from improving quality to patient safety. Too many physicians believe that in the patient safety arena, the hospital administration is the leader. Hospital administrators, at the same time, have had their own default position when it comes to safety and quality. They often believe they can't do anything that would upset physicians, who are viewed as the revenue generators in the system. Hospital administrators have tended to tiptoe around physicians.

So there has been a paradox at the heart of patient safety and quality. Physicians claim to be the captains of the ship and then miss the opportunity for leadership in patient safety. Hospital administrators claim to be leaders but abdicate responsibility for leading because their actions might upset physicians. So who, then, is in charge?

Add to these problems another one. In many institutions, like our own, hospital leadership seems ready to tackle safety and quality. So are some physicians. But to really address this problem, we have to have every physician on board, which means not only physicians who work in the hospital and clinics but also those involved in the educational mission of the medical school. We also have to enlist other professions and occupations.

Because of the complexity of the problems I have outlined, we realized that quick fixes would not work and that only through a sustained and organized effort could we change culture. We also recognized that we would need help, both to recruit physician leaders and other professional leaders and in guidance for structuring our culture-change process.

As a physician leader in this effort, I recognized that I, like so many other MDs, had not been taught the skills needed to lead teams, analyze culture, and create behavioral and attitudinal change throughout an institution. I thus contacted the Wharton School of Business of the University of Pennsylvania, where the management researcher Sigal Barsade is an international expert on emotional intelligence and organizational behavior. She suggested that we begin by conducting an organizational-affect survey that would help us understand the makeup of our current culture. With her help and that of her colleagues we designed a survey for the entire medical center so that we could measure our current cognitive and emotional culture.

By doing this we hoped to accomplish three things. First, we could discover our baseline so that we could measure the effectiveness of any culture-change intervention we designed and implemented. Second, we wanted to know if there were different cultural attitudes in the two distinct entities that make up our medical center. Are the medical school and hospital alike or different in our cognitive focus—the way we look at respect for others, teamwork, and innovation? On the emotional level, we wanted to know, as the patient safety physician Lucian Leape and his colleagues at the National Patient Safety Foundation have asked, do we have cultures of love and joy in our institutions, or are our workplaces filled with people who are angry, fearful, and sad?[8] The answers to these questions would help us accomplish our third goal, which was to gain the kind of insight needed to design the right kind of interventions.

We sent our survey out to 2,950 people in the medical school and hospital, and 1,711 responded to it. Overall, we had a response rate of 58 percent. We discovered that there is very little, if any, difference between those in the medical school and hospital with respect to cognitive and emotional cultural values. People in both institutions say they highly value respect for other people and that they value teamwork. When asked about love and joy at work, respondents said they wanted to care for their patients and one another but, in both institutions, their anger, fear, sadness, envy, loneliness, and guilt were stronger drivers than feelings of love and joy.

What creates this paradox? Studies have suggested that this kind of anger and frustration stems from feelings of injustice and thwarted goals. In their comments, many people said they felt blocked from achieving their goals or were frustrated because they couldn't get things done. They also expressed sadness and fear and added that they had given up and felt helpless. Superiors were commonly the primary source of their sense of helplessness and fear in the institution. In fact, people sometimes felt a threat to their survival at a corporate level. Again, the literature suggests that these threats frequently stem from their superiors. Clearly, it is difficult to create genuine teamwork in such an environment.

After analyzing this data we formed a culture-change steering committee composed of eight leaders from our medical center representing physicians, nurses, clinic operations, finance, and the Dean's Office. Our goal is to design interventions that decrease the anger, fear, and sadness in our medical school so that the beneficial components of our culture flourish. One of the interventions we are working on is a coordinated communication plan about patient safety initiatives so that we launch initiatives in a thoughtful and effective way.

At this writing, we are at the beginning of what we realize will be a long journey. Changing the many cultures in a truly multicultural institution that employs about three thousand people who work in various capacities and come from different backgrounds with varying educational backgrounds and individual professional and occupational expectations and expertise will take years, a minimum of five if not longer. But this is a journey that must be taken.

· · ·

FRANCIS A. ROSINIA, MD is an Associate Professor and Chairman of the Department of Anesthesiology and Chief Quality Officer at Tulane University where he practices anesthesiology. He sits on several national quality boards for Anesthesiology and is the author of several book chapters on publications on patient safety and practice management.

Going Live with Teaching Teamwork

Jason Adelman

As the patient safety officer at Montefiore Medical Center in the Bronx, I cover four hospitals with 1,500 beds and forty-six operating rooms across all our facilities. Operating rooms are a site of both promise and peril, depending on the safety protocols and measures taken during surgical operations. My job as patient safety officer is to eliminate the perils and enhance the promise of surgery.

In the case of my current work at Montefiore, the story starts with the Joint Commission and its Universal Protocol, whose goal is to prevent errors in the OR. There are three components to the Universal Protocol—conducting a preoperative checklist to make sure the surgeon has everything needed for surgery (e.g., implants or special surgical equipment), marking the surgical site so that there are no wrong-site surgeries, and finally a time-out immediately preceding the procedure before any incision is made. The time-out is just what it says—the surgical team stops right before the first incision to do a final check and make sure they have the right patient, right procedure, and are on the correct side of the body when laterality is an issue. The surgeon marks the site with his or her initials, and not with an *X*, because an *X* can be misinterpreted to mean "not this side."

As patient safety officer one of my core responsibilities is to make sure the organization is compliant with the Joint Commission national patient safety goals and regulations including the Universal Protocol. These include not only Joint Commission requirements but also New York state regulations including the New York State Surgical and Invasive Procedure Protocol, which is very similar to the Joint Commission's Universal Protocol.

While I was working on compliance with these safety measures, I began to realize that there is really no evidence to support that the utilization of the Universal Protocol actually prevents errors. It certainly makes sense, but it is not evidenced based. What we do have is evidence that using the World Health Organization checklist and teamwork decreases harm in the operating room. The leading research on the use of checklists and teamwork in the operating room was done by Dr. Atul Gawande and Dr. Jim Bagian, the physician-astronaut who brought the principles of teamwork used by NASA and the military to the VA when he was the chief patient safety officer for the Veterans Health Administration.[9]

With this research in mind, I decided to work not just on the Universal Protocol but also on implementing the WHO checklist and build teamwork skills into our operating rooms. I was convinced that doing all of this was not only complementary but also created a much stronger edifice for patient safety. However, there were a few obstacles to overcome. The first was resources. I received a $30,000 grant from Cardinal Healthcare to implement the WHO checklist and teamwork together. Our effort was further supported when Montefiore became a site in an Agency for Healthcare Research and Quality study regarding malpractice and patient safety. To launch our effort, I invited Dr. Bagian to meet with senior leadership and speak with staff about the merits of teamwork. I also bought two thousand copies of Atul Gawande's *Checklist Manifesto* and distributed them to all OR staff. In addition, I made large copies of our version of the WHO checklist, which we adapted—or "Montefiorized"—by adding and removing a few elements to match our work flows. We then displayed them in all the operating rooms in our four hospitals.

In addition to implementing the WHO checklist, we made plans to roll out the Agency for Health Care Research and Quality Team-STEPPS program to all perioperative services including surgeons, the Anesthesia Department, Nursing, Central Sterile Processing, and others.[10] Several months into the preparations, our plans were enhanced when our insurance carrier, FOJP, began rolling out their initiatives regarding surgical safety and required that all of their hospitals do the TeamSTEPPS training for all OR staff.

The trick to successfully rolling out a program such as Team-STEPPS, as with any patient safety initiative, is to get buy-in from both senior leadership as well as frontline staff. Without this kind of buy-in, you don't have the right synergy, and initiatives that could be promising and lead to change become little more than pro forma box-checking exercises. To make sure TeamSTEPPS had a real impact in daily practice and to develop a robust education plan, we created a leadership team made up of the hospital's chief learning officer, Dr. Helen Slaven, who oversees the Learning Network with roughly twenty FTEs working in it; the patient safety manager, Amisha Rai; and the chief of General Surgery and chief quality officer, Dr. Peter Shamamian. The four of us then went on to create a larger steering committee that met every other week to engage other leaders in the perioperative services. The membership of this steering group included the vice president of OR Services, the director of nursing for Surgery, the chair of Anesthesia, the vice chairman of Orthopedic Surgery, and a senior physician from Obstetrics/Gynecology, who had already lead a TeamSTEPPS initiative on the Labor and Delivery unit.

We discussed a lot of ways to effectively teach TeamSTEPPS. We decided to begin with an off-site retreat for those who would eventually become our TeamSTEPPS "coaches." About fifty leaders from across all of Montefiore's ORs met at a hotel in Rye, New York, for a day-and-a-half retreat funded by FOJP. Nurses, physicians (surgeons and anesthesiologists), OR technicians, and administrators all went through a fourteen-hour TeamSTEPPS curriculum in which the core TeamSTEPPS skills were taught. In multiple group discussions, participants brainstormed on how to effectively teach this to the rest of their 1,500 operating room colleagues. Given the quantity of people across different disciplines and multiple campuses, the question remained, "How do we do it?" We decided to divide the curriculum into four ninety-minute modules covering the main TeamSTEPPS concepts.

At Montefiore, Monday is our late OR start day, which means that rather than beginning to operate at 7 a.m., we start at 9 a.m. The preceding hours are usually reserved for grand rounds. Because of the importance of this initiative and the emphasis from leadership, all the surgical subspecialties and anesthesia agreed that we could replace grand rounds with TeamSTEPPs on the third Monday in the month for four consecutive months. At each of these Monday sessions, we discussed one of the following topics: leadership, situation monitoring, teamwork, and communication.

Our surgeon-in-chief, Dr. Robert Michler, presented the very first session on leadership. A cardiothoracic transplant surgeon, Dr. Michler is chairman of cardiothoracic surgery in addition to overseeing all of the surgical subspecialties. As an avid sailor he also brought his perspective of teamwork and leadership involved in sailing and related the concepts to the operating room. While Dr. Michler was presenting in one lecture hall, we used video technology to simulcast to five other conference rooms all across Montefiore, including two hospitals miles away. In addition to the simulcast, we had separate video cameras taping him so we could reuse the session at other venues and for new associates in the future. After a half-hour discussion, a leader in each room facilitated an interactive conversation with participants.

Although the session was a big success, the video conferencing had technical difficulties and did not go as well as we had hoped. The screen went dark a couple of times; the sound wasn't as loud as we wanted it to be; and it was hard to see the presenter and slides at the same time. These technical issues had to be addressed. To do this, we decided that we would videotape the speaker who would present the next topic ahead of time, which allowed us to show the same session in all locations at the same time. Interspersed within the presentations were video clips of funny commercials or scenarios that highlighted a particular point and added some entertainment to prevent a boring PowerPoint or lecture format. The presenters included surgeons and anesthesiologists from Montefiore and FOJP who were experts in TeamSTEPPS.

To keep each session interactive, we split each speaker video into five to ten minute segments, followed by thought-provoking questions to stimulate discussion among the participants. To get the most out of the group discussions, a live moderator at each site led the discussion, facilitated the group, and provided real-time feedback. The moderators included several senior surgeons, an anesthesiologist, and a physician assistant who were all at our TeamSTEPPS retreat. In addition, each room had several staff from the Learning Network who would help facilitate the conversation between the moderator and the audience.

What we learned is that using prerecorded videos worked out well. It proved to be more reliable, engaging, and allowed us better control of the format and content. That model made the remaining three sessions more successful. After every session we had a round of makeup sessions for those who couldn't attend. We went to each campus and gave the talk three more times using the prerecorded videos. We were not quite at 100 percent attendance so we decided to repurpose the videos into an e-learning module that was accessible from any Montefiore computer and even home.

At the end of this journey, we had instilled the basic language and core concepts of TeamSTEPPS throughout the entire operating room staff. The next step is to monitor performance in the operating rooms and answer the forever-challenging question, "How do we operationalize these concepts and make them sustainable?" In the preliminary stages of planning for sustainability we wanted to encourage the frontline staff of each subspecialty to take ownership of different concepts that they thought were most important in their area. We conducted an Innovation Tournament where about thirty leaders were present to generate ideas with a winning idea from each campus that the team would be tasked to complete. To guide the group, three larger themes were communicated: (1) achieving improved OR efficiency through teamwork, (2) identifying and managing OR emergencies, and (3) improving safety by driving utilization of core TeamSTEPPS skills.

Through this journey we have learned a lot about the operating room setting and challenges within this high-acuity area, which has further highlighted the benefit of teamwork. Although we have achieved a lot through this process, we recognize that there is still much work to be done.

· · ·

JASON ADELMAN, MD is the Patient Safety Officer at Montefiore Medical Center, a large integrated health care delivery system in the Bronx, and the University Hospital for the Albert Einstein College of Medicine. He is a member of the National Quality Forum (NQF) Committee on Patient Safety Complications, on the editorial boards of the *Journal for Healthcare Quality* and the National Patient Safety Foundation's *Insight* magazine, and was named one of "fifty experts leading the field of patient safety" by Becker's *Hospital Review*.

The Change in Rwanda

Jessica Early

In late May 2013, after a day spent napping off the jet lag from my transatlantic multiple-layover journey from Boston to Rwanda, I found myself sitting in a plastic lawn chair squeezed into a small medical exam room at the Women's Equity in Access to Care and Treatment (WE-ACTx) clinic in Kigali. It was my first day as a volunteer nurse at this community health initiative, founded in 2004 by foreign and domestic HIV/AIDS patients, activists, and physicians. Today, the organization provides medical and psychosocial care to HIV-infected men, women, and children. On this particular morning, I was the only foreign volunteer working at its Kigali facility, which serves over 1,800 patients. The clinic is staffed entirely by Rwandans working in interdisciplinary teams of medical and psychosocial workers.

These staff members welcomed me with a flurry of high fives, smiles, and kisses. Despite their warm reception, I was filled with apprehension when the exam room door closed behind me, heralding the arrival of my first patient. As a young, newly licensed RN, I would only be observing and assisting Jane, my middle-aged white-coat-clad fellow nurse, but the idea that I might be making a contribution to a patient's clinical care plan and the health care team of nurses, doctors, and psychosocial counselors seemed far-fetched.

During my clinical rotations in nursing school, I had cared for only one or two HIV-positive patients. So, in a frantic bid to alleviate feelings of anxiety and professional inadequacy, I had spent weeks prior to my trip reading medical journal articles, global health studies, and, I must admit, Wikipedia entries on the transmission, pathophysiology, clinical presentation, and treatment of HIV and AIDS. In a small notebook, I had scrawled "cheat sheets" of CD4 count-based treatment algorithms, common side effects of antiretrovirals (ARVs), and the signs and symptoms of an array of opportunistic infections.

By immersing myself in as much HIV- and AIDS-related research as possible, I naively hoped that I could compensate for my near-total lack of practical experience working with HIV-infected patients.

When Jane's first patient walked into the exam room, I kept my little notebook of factoids and protocols close at hand. Drawing on my mastery of about ten words in Kinyarwanda, I greeted this forty-something Rwandan woman who was dressed in a traditional wrap skirt and matching blouse. Jane asked the patient how she was doing, and the two launched into an animated discussion in Kinyarwanda that I could not understand at all.

Instead, while awaiting Jane's translation, I tried to put my skills of inspection—the first step in the physical assessment, which had been drilled into my head in nursing school—to good use. I scanned the patient's skin from head to toe searching for rashes, discolorations, hair loss, and evidence of dermatological infections. Watching the subtle rise and fall of the patient's chest, I determined her respiratory rate and looked for any signs of labored breathing. After making a gross estimation of the patient's height and weight, I calculated her body mass index as falling somewhere in the low end of the overweight range.

Finally, I observed the patient's facial expressions, vocal intonations, and mannerisms as she chatted away with Jane. Opening up to a blank page of my notebook, I jotted down my initial clinical impression: "Middle-aged, overweight Rwandan female alert and oriented times three in no acute distress. Appropriate eye contact, dress, and speech pattern with pleasant affect." I silently reread my assessment a few times and found myself immediately perplexed with her as a patient:

The red, itchy patches of cutaneous Candidiasis that prey on immunocompromised skin? *Negative.*

Hollow cheeks and atrophied limbs from malnourishment or HIV-wasting syndrome? *The woman sitting in front of me is pleasantly plump.*

Signs and symptoms of cytomegalovirus (CMV), *Pneumocystis jirovecii* pneumonia (PCP), or histoplasmosis? *Not present.*

In short, where was the presentation of an HIV-positive patient living in a developing East African nation that all my pretrip research had described?

Before even hearing her reason for coming in, I suspected I would not find a portrait of this patient among my research notes. When Jane translated the chief complaint as hot flashes and moodiness, my suspicion was confirmed. In a country with limited resources, immense population pressure, and a recent history of genocide and subsequent economic collapse, and where I thought I would surely encounter clinical presentations and illnesses rarely seen in the United States, I formulated my first likely diagnosis: menopause.

WE-ACTx has spent the past decade tirelessly promoting patient adherence to therapeutic regimens and self-management of HIV through a multimodal and totally team-based approach to care that includes individual and group psychosocial counseling, peer-to-peer patient education, nutrition assistance, income-generation projects, and targeted support programs for children and young adults. In its early years—when ARVs were just becoming available in Rwanda—much of WE-ACTx's work was directed at facilitating access to HIV treatment. Faced with a patient population experiencing rapid disease progression and resulting immune system failure and opportunistic infections, WE-ACTx's priority was getting patients on life-saving drugs.

Today, the Rwandan government provides ARVs for free through a network of private and public clinics. Moreover, WE-ACTx's provider-patient partnerships have markedly increased adherence to these drugs. As a result of these collaborations, the clinic can devote more energy and resources toward primary care alongside HIV-specific treatment. Patients receive care for and learn how to manage medical and psychosocial issues from hypertension and diabetes to depression and domestic or interpersonal conflicts. From an organization urgently providing ARVs at a time when patients were succumbing to the disease every day, WE-ACTx has evolved into a primary care provider that addresses the holistic needs of its patients and supports their efforts to improve their overall quality of life as people living with HIV—not dying of AIDS.

Which brings me back to my first patient encounter. I was looking at the new face of HIV care at WE-ACTx: a rotund, chatty, middle-aged Rwandan woman who was fatigued not by an opportunistic infection ravaging her immunocompromised body but rather by a night spent tossing and turning, sweating, and stripping off her clothes as an uncomfortable wave of heat spread over her torso and left her face flushed.

None of the ARVs I had so frantically researched would relieve the menopausal symptoms suffered by this patient and numerous others I later met who were experiencing "the change" during my visit to Rwanda. In their country, hormone replacement therapy—whose utility and safety remains controversial in the United States—is available from just a handful of prohibitively expensive specialists in private practice. Jane and I could only offer reassurance that these hot flashes, while distressing and disruptive, were a classic sign of a natural, inevitable physical and emotional transition rather than a harbinger of disease.

We also encouraged our middle-aged patient to discuss her experience at her weekly WE-ACTx women's support group meeting, a safe space for sharing medical, familial, and socioeconomic struggles and successes. At this session, her "treatment" would take the form of knowing smiles, nodding heads, words of commiseration, and copious amounts of laughter from fellow peri- or postmenopausal patients. Just a few years ago, this same group of patients had little hope of even reaching middle age and thus being able to experience this natural condition.

In my first encounter with menopause in Rwanda (and in many other patient appointments to come), I did not deploy an arsenal of differential diagnoses or drug options. Instead, I had a far more educational opportunity to participate in the type of interdisciplinary patient-centered holistic care—increasingly uncommon in the profit-driven US health system—that all patients deserve, whether in a small, developing East African country or the wealthiest nation in the world.

• • •

JESSICA EARLY, RN, Family Nurse Practitioner, is a graduate of the Yale School of Nursing masters program.

The Devil's in the Details

Loraine O'Neill

My nursing education in a London teaching hospital in the early 1970s afforded me the opportunity to practice in a collaborative care model. As a team, the nurses and doctors walked the wards (yes, in true Florence Nightingale fashion) stopping at each patient's bedside to review the individual's current status and plan of care. As the primary nurse, I was expected to know everything about my patient from medications to labs to dietary needs, and my part of the briefing process was to go over how my patients were doing. In this way I was hardwired for team function and performance.

Fast forward almost thirty years to my current job as director of quality and safety for the Obstetrics and Gynecology Department in a large academic medical center in the US Northeast. In this role I have been trained in the aviation-safety model known as crew resource management. I have taken two different courses in health care team training based on this model. Regardless of which model is adopted—and there are several—the primary focus of such methods is to ensure that team function becomes embedded in daily practice requiring "stick-to-it-ism."

In my most recent foray into facilitating teamwork, we have adapted the training developed by the Agency for Healthcare Research and Quality and Department of Defense called TeamSTEPPS. After attending TeamSTEPPS training, our group of thirteen nurses and physicians returned to the hospital ready to forge ahead with what we agreed would be our first step—improving communication. It is easy to state that we were going to improve the way in which we talk to our medical and other colleagues, but the truth is that this is very complex. We needed to coach, give feedback, recoach, and support staff for several months to see an improvement and full assimilation of Situation-Background-Assessment-Recommendation (SBAR) and other techniques into our daily contacts and handovers.

SBAR is a technique that is now used in health care to communicate information in an effective way. To give one example, a nurse calling a physician about a patient would introduce herself to the physician and present the patient situation (S): "My name is Loraine O'Neill. I am the registered nurse taking care of Mrs. Smith, and she's bleeding"; the background (B): "She just had a vacuum delivery with blood loss of 400 ccs thirty minutes ago. She was on Pitocin in labor for over fifteen hours"; the assessment (A): "Her blood pressure is 120/80, and her pulse is 80. Her uterus is boggy, but she is not passing any clots"; and a Recommendation (R): "Could you please come and assess her?" Although we taught the SBAR technique to everyone on the unit, we realized that patient safety involved more than one person giving the information via SBAR to another member of the team. The individual receiving the information had to repeat back what was heard so it was clear that everyone was on the same page with understanding the information conveyed. The SBAR at handoff required closing the loop in this way—ensuring that peers were not only given information but that they were engaged and actively listening. We also realized that a shorter SBAR was required in emergency situations. For example, "I have nonreassuring tracings in Room 34. I need you there now." To make sure that the primary care provider—either physician or midwife—actually made it to the room, everyone had to be taught this shorthand and to respond to it immediately.

But again, what might look straightforward is actually more involved. The difficulty here is that the nurse's immediate need for the physician or midwife might interrupt other urgent work that the physician is engaged in. Therefore, we had to learn how to specifically request the time frame involved, because "immediately" could mean right now or in ten minutes. What might seem like a small detail is extremely important in a large institution where someone might be engaged in an activity on another floor and therefore can't respond immediately to a request. In health care the pattern has been that someone requests help and someone else doesn't clearly say, "No, I can't do it!" Instead, they tend to say, "I'll be there soon." But their "soon" might be in half an hour when they are needed in two minutes. But if the nurse knew they couldn't come "immediately"—as in two minutes—they could find someone else who could. The person being asked to clarify the time frame would often get irritated or offended: "What does 'now' mean? I'm in the middle of examining a patient." If someone is in the middle of examining a patient she or he won't be able to help for another ten or fifteen minutes, which a nurse needs to know. Now, as we have repeated the training and conducted a lot of coaching, people have finally become accustomed to defining when *exactly* they will be available. As they always say, the devil is in the details, and applying team training effectively means teasing out those details and adjusting the tool to the local culture.

Another thing that we needed to address was psychological safety. In order to carry out effective team training and implement teamwork people have to know that they can speak up and that doing so won't be held against them. When I started working on perinatal safety, I was taught to "till the soil" before attempting to implement any changes in practice. To me this has meant speaking with, observing, and working with a group before moving to educate them. As a person who loves to watch people this has not been difficult for me. Therefore, the first thing we did before helping to implement Team-STEPPS was to hold focus groups with the various groups, obstetricians and midwives as well as the nurses and neonatologists, about their comfort level with using the tools we were providing such as SBAR or the "two-challenge rule," which is used to challenge another colleague about an unsafe practice. In these sessions, a nurse might say, "Well, I won't be able to say that to Dr. So-and-so." Then what you have to do is see if their peers have ideas of how to deal with that particular physician. Or you may have to reiterate to the group that every member of the team is going to have to learn important language that will enable them to stop the line to insure that everyone adheres to rules of patient safety. So now we use the words, "I need clarity."

If there is an issue with Dr. X in the delivery room where the patient is always awake, the nurse can say, "I need clarity," which is a signal to stop what the team is doing and then, if it's safe, move out of the room and have a private conversation about the issue at hand. If things don't work out and it regards patient safety, we would then invoke the chain of command. After doing this work for the past four years, we have never had a serious escalation of a problem. What we have found instead is that often people are just so focused on what they need to do that they ignore their teammates' concerns. When, through using some of the techniques described above, their focus is broken, they realize that a patient safety issue that has been raised by a colleague needs an appropriate response.

It is worth repeating that this doesn't happen without a lot of education that is delivered multiple times. You can say you have taught your whole health care system team training, but if you have simply presented information to people, it doesn't automatically move people from ingrained patterns of behavior to new ones. You have to have the processes in place, but you also have to have champions and coaches who are available day and night. You have to post their telephone numbers. You have to make sure that the coaches respond appropriately to such phone calls for help or guidance, because the first time someone calls for help and has their head bitten off, that's the end of your system.

These telephone numbers that are posted mostly come from those in leadership positions. Their buy-in to these safety practices is essential. Our chairman once took a call from a postpartum nurse while on the golf course. He was very receptive, and the nurse obviously passed this along to her peers. When the chairman next visited that unit for safety rounds the nurse and he had a long discussion about the call, the outcome of his intervention, and (naturally) how his golf game went.

Working in a busy obstetrical unit can be highly challenging. We have always been able to pull together, particularly in extreme emergences such as a cord prolapse or an abruption, a massive bleed before the delivery of a baby. Now, with these new safety tools under our belt, we have considerably fewer adverse outcomes. However, we are all human. So, when my colleagues start to begin criticizing and bemoaning circumstances, I remind them that we are privileged to come to work every day to help a family through a life-changing event—namely, childbirth. My motto is "It is all for the patient."

. . .

LORAINE O'NEILL, RN trained and practiced as a nurse and midwife in the United Kingdom. She has worked in the field of Obstetrics from administration to research and now in quality and safety. She holds an MPH from the Mailman School of Public Health, Columbia University. She lives and works in New York City.

Walking the Walk

Pamela Brier

For as long as I've been a hospital CEO, I've known that you need a supportive work environment for staff if you expect them to take good care of patients. I also know that leading efforts to change behavior in hospitals isn't easy. When you're trying to create a supportive work environment—especially when it comes to patient safety—many managers will insist that staff are valued members of the health care team and encourage them to speak up and alert others to unsafe practices. Yet, when nurses, residents, housekeepers, and others do just what they are exhorted to do, they feel that they are unsupported. This is a problem in every hospital.

At Maimonides, we've tried over the years to encourage people to speak up about patient care problems and let them know that they'll be protected when they do so. The real issue for us has been having managers see and acknowledge the problem. When someone reports a problem, a manager might say, "What are you talking about? That doesn't happen here." And so the person who raises the problem or issue is shut down.

This occurs because it's difficult to support and engage staff at every level of the hospital. Vice presidents who report to me and assistant vice presidents who report to them may understand that a supportive work environment is important. This doesn't mean, however, that our middle managers—people I might not meet with on a day-to-day basis—understand they are expected to create an environment where staff actively participates in improving their workplace. If we want to have teamwork that supports patient safety and quality care, it can't be top down with managers just giving orders. They have to get workers engaged in the work. Working in teams—communicating and feeling respected—is important not just because it's a nice thing to do but because it's a smart thing to do.

Logistically, this is very hard. At Maimonides, we now have fifteen labor-management committees, one in every major unit. Our goal is to get people throughout the hospital feeling connected to their work, to have an opportunity to improve their work and working conditions, and to be respected in the process. We want everyone who works here to be involved in making the hospital a better place. So we're trying to make that happen by raising staff engagement as a strategic priority, rewarding success, and training managers to operate in this way.

We try to give our managers the tools they need to be successful. This means, for example, teaching people things like how to run a meeting so that everyone feels free to talk. It means that it's not okay for managers to dictate how things operate on a top-down basis. It really is not. So, it's my job to continually engage senior staff in this so that people know that I'm serious.

Of course, the best way to make managers engage with their staff is to incorporate it into their performance review. It's taken us a while to figure this out because you need an effective way to do it—but people certainly pay attention to their evaluations. After telling managers for years that we expect this, we are now going to be looking at data from a staff-engagement survey to make this determination. We're still working this out, but we want to measure whether staff feel connected to their work.

Another fundamental issue for me is leading by example. This means making it clear that respect is a fundamental aspect of the organization. It is important that people understand they will be protected and supported even when—at times—they are disrespected by high-ranking people—for example, by physicians who generate a great deal of revenue for the hospital.

At Maimonides Medical Center, our medical staff instituted a standard we call the Code of Mutual Respect that must be signed by every physician who comes to work here. It has structured and progressive steps to deal with someone who is consistently disrespectful. When the code was introduced, I spoke at the staff meeting and said that I would enforce the code and that nobody was exempt. No one. I explained that nobody brings in so much money or is so important that they are permitted to behave disrespectfully—nobody.

After I made this statement, everybody applauded. But I am sure that many people really thought, "Oh yeah, right!"

However, I was determined that we could show people that we were serious about respect in our institution. The Code of Mutual Respect involves conversation, coaching, and progressive discipline. If there are reports of disrespect in which there is a problem between two people, we bring them together with a facilitator. If problems continue and people are reported five times—even voluntary physicians who are privileged and admit patients—then they just can't work here anymore. We have taken this kind of action—mostly with doctors who have not behaved respectfully time and time again. As I said in that first meeting, no one is that good that they can behave in a way that jeopardizes teamwork and mutual respect. It's too important to patient safety.

We've also shown that we are serious by allocating significant resources to trainings in our departments on "respect intervention tools" such as Crucial Conversations. We have trained doctors to staff hotlines and others to be keepers of this kind of conflict resolution. Today, anyone who has an experience with bad physician behavior can call the hotline. We have also focused on particular units, such as perioperative services, with structured programs such as TeamSTEPPS, and we follow up with coaching and mentoring.

Finally, when real-life problems occur, we also have to be prepared to take action. For example, on one unit, we discovered that, although they had not raised it much with management, nurses were upset because the unit had a large, well-appointed physician lounge, while the nurses' lounge was tiny and looked terrible. The nurses felt really bad about that. So what to do?

The leaders of this service got together and said, "Well, why don't we have everybody use the same lounge?" A senior physician objected to this. So I said, "Why don't we just fix up the nurses' lounge and turn that into something else, like an area for charting and then share the other lounge? This way everybody gets a little something." That's what we are doing.

The take-home message here is that you've got to be creative and look for opportunities to make the operations consistent with the message we are preaching. Issues like this may seem petty when compared with larger problems of patient safety, but they have great significance for the people they affect. You can't really be teaching TeamSTEPPS and talk about people working together if one group has a nice setup and the other group has not much at all. That's not practicing what we are preaching. As CEO, I have to get the message out that we are serious about what we are saying.

Changing culture and how people behave is slow and difficult work. The question that always arises is, "How do you know that you are making progress?" Some time ago, we did a survey throughout the hospital that asked people, "Do you respect others?" Of course, everyone said, "Yes." However, when asked whether they get respect, the answer came back, "Not so much." After launching the initiatives I just discussed, we did a follow-up survey in perioperative services and found that people felt that they were working in an environment that was more respectful and that things had improved. It is slow and difficult work, and it is never complete. You just have to keep at it.

· · ·

PAMELA BRIER is the President and Chief Executive Officer of Maimonides Medical Center. She has been at Maimonides since 1995, for eight years as Executive Vice President/Chief Operating Officer and since 2003 as the leader of this major teaching hospital. She currently serves as Vice Chair of the Board of the New York eHealth Collaborative (NYeC), a statewide public/private partnership organization devoted to health IT promulgation and adoption. She also serves on the City's Board of Corrections and is a board member of the Fund for Public Health in New York City.

Medical Teamwork Is All That Jazz

Theresa Brown

I was getting an admission from the Emergency Department. She'd been in an irregular heart rhythm—atrial fibrillation—and they said she'd converted, or returned to, a normal rhythm on her own. I knew the conversion might not be permanent, and sure enough, when she got on the floor she was back in a fib and her heart rate was jumping between 140 and 160.

I could have called in a rapid response team, but my sense was that she didn't need that level of reaction. Her heart rate was high, and she felt lousy, but she wasn't really in distress. What she did need was coordinated effort to get her stabilized.

And, somewhat unusually, that's what ended up happening. Her medical intern and resident came over and waited, watching her heart rhythm on the cardiac monitor while I administered the drugs they ordered. I was supposed to get another extra patient, but seeing what I was tied up with, another nurse took that patient for me. The nursing student I was training made sure the other patients we were taking care of were covered.

It took more than an hour to convert our patient, but when we were done she felt normal again. The other patients on the floor had gotten the care they needed, and best of all, the annoying ding of the heart monitor alarm was silent.

That silence was music to our ears. And although medicine and music are typically thought of as very different endeavors, while watching a jazz concert in Pittsburgh in fall 2011, and thinking back on this patient in a fib, I realized that modern health care could learn some important lessons about teamwork and collegiality from jazz musicians. Improvisation matters in jazz of course, and health care is a lot about thinking on your feet. But a marked absence of ego in performance, combined with visible demonstrations of professional respect and appreciation, are the ideas that health care could beneficially adopt from jazz.

The concert I attended was the culminating event of the Jazz Seminar and Concert that the University of Pittsburgh organizes every year. Jazz greats from all over the country come together to spend one evening making standout music in a packed Pittsburgh auditorium.

I went with my husband, and because he's the musician, not I, I found myself studying how the musicians worked as a group. I didn't evaluate their technique—because I don't have the expertise to do that—but acted as a sociologist, observing how these ten musicians who'd never played together before collaborated to make an amazing musical event.

Collaboration is a requirement for any individuals who want to play music together. The Jazz Concert at the University of Pittsburgh revealed jazz to me as a standout example, even among musical groupings, of truly collaborative music making. The three traits of jazz music that for me exemplify its collaborative nature are the leader's role is subtle; appreciation for a job well done is built into the performances; and most of the time the musicians have to subordinate their egos to the musical needs of the piece being performed.

It took me thirty minutes of pretty careful watching to figure out who was in charge of the jazz group at the Pittsburgh concert. Nathan Davis, a saxophonist, was the leader of the group, but he stood in line with the other brass players, was dressed like everyone else, and rarely made an obvious signal as to who would play next or even what they would play. He kept time by snapping the fingers of his right hand close to his right leg, and he would casually point at players during each piece to indicate who would perform the next solo. It was elegant, unobtrusive leadership, even though Davis, a PhD musician, is a world-famous jazzer and director of Jazz Studies at the University of Pittsburgh. Davis could have commanded the stage, but he didn't; he was the musical leader of the group, but he was very much part of the group, too.

This practice of seeing every musician as an integral part of the group was complemented by the musicians' habit of showing appreciation for each other's performances. Whenever a player finished a solo—whether on trombone, piano, or bass—the other players would smile, energetically nod their heads, and if they were close enough, high five the soloist. Additionally, if players could, they made space for soloists by walking to the back edges of the stage. When Randy Brecker, a young trumpet player, did his astounding riffs, the other brass players hovered at the periphery, nodding their heads. Every soloist was allowed to enjoy time in the spotlight, and only when solos neared their end did other musicians wander back to the center of the stage, ready for the next combined blast of musical effort.

Keep this image of the jazz concert in your head as we move back to health care, imagining morning rounds in a hospital. The rounding team, consisting of an attending physician accompanied by subordinate interns, residents, fellows, nurse practitioners, and physician assistants, goes into the patient's room. The nurse may or may not be there. When nurses are not at rounds it's usually because they don't know the team is rounding on their patient or because they don't have time.

In the patient's room the attending physician does a brief physical exam, explains how the treatment is going, and asks in a more or less cursory manner, depending on the doctor and on how much time she has, if the patient has any questions. Then the team leaves, moving as quickly as possible to the next patient.

If the nurse, the person who will take care of the patient for the next twelve hours, has missed rounds, then she will not be much help in answering the patient's further questions. Also, if the patient got definitive news or needs to have a scan done or labs drawn, the nurse won't know until the interns and residents take time to explain it to the RN or have time to put in orders. Additionally, the other members of the medical team might have had questions or comments that the attending physician didn't have time to address or, in the cases of particularly willful attendings, wasn't willing to entertain.

I'm not so naive as to say that modern health care should be run like a jazz concert. Trying to restore health on a 24/7 schedule is more complicated than spending a couple hours making great music, but looking at how jazz musicians play with and for each other provides a thought-provoking example of egoless collaborative work. Jazz shows that for true collaboration to occur everyone must be expected and allowed to contribute.

That is exactly what happened when we were treating my patient with a fib. The resident was in charge, but only insofar as he had to decide on orders and explain his clinical decisions to his intern. My solo came when I gave the IV drugs ordered by the doctor, talked with the patient to evaluate how she was doing, and kept track of her vitals, making sure she remained stable. The nurse who took my extra patient was making her own beautiful music, and my nursing student kept time—making sure all of our patients were okay while I kept busy taking care of this one woman.

Morning rounds, in contrast, are usually a fairly static clinical situation, and that's why I suggest it is a time and place to start giving collaboration in health care the jazz treatment. Rounds are the ideal place for attending physicians to model collaborative practice. Interns and residents are learning how to be doctors, and they should be allowed to ask questions and share opinions and to speak as colleagues rather than subordinates to become the best doctors possible for this new era of team medicine.

Not having the nurse at morning rounds is like trying to play jazz without a bass player. The nurse holds the patient's day together, keeps it moving at the right pace and in the right direction. A bass player may not stand out in a jazz group, but the absence of that reliable rhythmic drive will be audibly noticeable, just as the absence of the nurse in rounds will make it that much harder to keep the patient's care on track.

A top-down model of decision making may seem to best suit the time demands of modern hospitals, and time is always of the essence in health care. But, even in hospitals, hierarchical leadership shouldn't have to mean that the leader is authoritarian, and as I saw in the jazz concert, only a leader who is determinedly unauthoritarian makes great collaboration possible. An attending physician who aggressively rejects input from the team—whether as a result of being pressed for time, impatient with having to share the stage during rounds, or both—will not get the best work out of the people charged with caring for the patient. Also, if medicine and nursing, and individual doctors and nurses, put more effort into appreciating one another's efforts—as jazz musicians do—we would have more personal incentive to truly work together.

The example of how my floor pulled together to take care of the patient in a fib ultimately shows how necessary teamwork is. If any one person in that situation had an overdeveloped sense of ego, or an underdeveloped commitment to all our patients, we would have had to call a rapid response team, maybe even send someone who wasn't that sick to ICU. None of that was necessary. We just needed a doctor who knew his meds and nurses who knew their jobs to give that patient the care she needed.

And, ultimately, the patient is the most important person in any discussion of how to improve health care. Getting patients better is the music we try to make in the hospital every day. Our melodies aren't always easy to tease out, and in the hardest cases sometimes we fall into cacophony, but the goal, always, is to produce harmony. That is, we want the patient to leave healed, or at least be on her or his way to recovery. To make our health care harmonies as dynamic, soulful, and effective as possible, we need to play with everyone chiming in, knowing that when we jam together we make the best music of all for patients.

· · ·

THERESA BROWN, RN, PhD is a staff nurse in Oncology and the author of *Critical Care: A New Nurse Faces Death, Life, and Everything in Between,* a memoir of her first year of nursing. Brown writes an opinion column, "Bedside," for the *New York Times.* In addition to her clinical and writing work, Brown is a member of the National Advisory Council for the Center for Health Media and Policy at Hunter College and a reviewer for and occasional contributor to *American Journal of Nursing.*

Investing in Meaningful, Sustainable Change

Carolyn Plummer and Joy Richards

There is an ancient and well-known story, turned into a poem by John Godfrey Saxe (1816–87), about six blind men and an elephant. The six blind men, in a quest to learn about and understand what the elephant was, approached it one by one—each encountering a different part and drawing conclusions about what the elephant resembled based on what he touched. For example, the man who touched the trunk concluded that elephants were like snakes; the man who touched a leg concluded that elephants were like trees; the man who touched an ear concluded that elephants were like fans. The men then engaged in a lengthy debate that led to conflict, each one convinced he was right; although there was some truth in what each of them found individually, no one man alone had a full understanding of what an elephant was.

The moral to this story is that the whole cannot be known or understood by only knowing or understanding its individual parts. Although there is truth and validity in differing perspectives, overall understanding is more likely when all perspectives are considered together. In the case of the blind men and the elephant, teamwork would have helped them to avoid conflict and achieve success in their quest.

Patient care can be looked at through a similar lens. Patient care does not belong to one specific individual, group, profession, department, or organization; patient care belongs to everyone in the system—and indeed, its very existence relies on the perspectives, contributions, and collaboration of all members of the team. In health care, good teamwork is a basic foundation for everyone to have a full understanding of what needs to happen to ensure the best care possible is provided for patients. It is also a basic foundation for evaluating and continually improving the way we do things.

Health professionals working at the point of care have many innovative ideas about ways to improve patient care. Acting on these ideas depends not only on being able to carry out research or quality-improvement initiatives but also on mobilizing teams with other health care providers and workers. Many of these health professionals, such as nurses or respiratory therapists, have historically found it difficult to initiate, participate in, or lead research or quality-improvement initiatives. The nature of their work, and the way it is organized, does not usually allow them the time to engage in work away from the point of care, especially in hospital settings. Other members of the team, such as physicians, have dedicated time in their schedules for—and are expected to engage in and lead—research and other projects, and they are evaluated (in part) on their contribution to research and quality-improvement efforts. Nurses and other point-of-care health professionals do not usually have this flexibility built into their day-to-day work schedules. They are, however, expected to engage in professional development activities. This generally involves ongoing individual learning about their practice (such as attending wound care training sessions or critical care conferences); the time and cost involved in this ongoing learning is often covered by the individual staff member. There is no formal expectation that nurses and others at the point of care lead or contribute to research and quality improvement—nor are they usually evaluated from this perspective. Without dedicated, protected time and institutional support, they are not able to turn their innovative ideas into action. This limits the impact that staff at the point of care can have on enhancing patient outcomes; it limits the contribution they can make to the team; and it limits critical thinking as these staff become focused on tasks rather than the bigger picture.

At University Health Network (UHN), we have found an innovative way to address this issue. UHN is a multisite academic health care organization in Toronto. It comprises four hospitals that are affiliated with the University of Toronto: Toronto General, Toronto Western, Toronto Rehab, and Princess Margaret Cancer Centre. In 2010, we developed and began implementing a grassroots initiative that is now called the Collaborative Academic Practice Innovation and Research Fellowship Program (CAP Fellowship Program). The CAP Fellowship Program provides an annual opportunity for point-of-care health professionals to lead an innovative quality-improvement or research project related to the organization's strategic priorities and to engage in ongoing dialogue and learning about leadership and leading change. All CAP Fellowship Program projects reflect "collaborative academic practice"—which is the synthesis of research, education, and practice to facilitate interprofessional collaboration, critical thinking, healthy work environments, and safe, patient-centered care. Participants engage their team members, patients and families, leaders, cross-organizational colleagues, other organizations, and current research evidence to help move their projects forward. The CAP Fellowship Program fosters curiosity at the point of care, empowers nurses and other health professionals to drive change, raises their organizational profile, liberates them from a task-oriented mindset, and helps strengthen their voice so they can have an impact on transformation of the health care system.

Interested health professionals submit comprehensive project proposals that are then rigorously reviewed by a selection committee made up of leaders in research, quality improvement, and interprofessional collaboration. Successful applicants are provided with paid protected time (two days per week for six months) for project completion as well as ongoing support from CAP leaders at UHN. The majority of the protected time is used to complete their CAP Fellowship Program projects; in addition, participants attend weekly seminars about leadership, change management, project management, interprofessional collaboration and teamwork, communication strategies, interprofessional knowledge-transfer strategies, and other topics.

The CAP Fellowship Program is intended for those staff members who would not ordinarily be able to leave their day-to-day work environment without coverage by other staff and who do not already have professional development or research time built into their roles. The CAP Fellowship Program began with nurses; it has now evolved to include other health professions. In the past four years, fifty-two point-of-care health professionals have participated; these include nurses, respiratory therapists, occupational and physical therapists, dietitians, speech-language pathologists, and kinesiologists. Their grassroots projects, which were inspired by critical questions they were asking in their day-to-day practice, address patient care and system issues with which health care leaders have struggled for decades (e.g., managing pain, preventing falls); through this program, participants have been able to achieve meaningful, sustainable change right at the point of care.

One example of a successful project of the CAP Fellowship Program is a joint initiative that was co-led by a registered nurse and a registered respiratory therapist. Their project involved developing an interprofessional education program to help clinical teams maintain and enhance their skills in code blue (cardiac arrest and resuscitation) situations. Historically, this training has been provided to individuals or to groups of staff from the same profession (e.g., groups of nurses) and has not included a teamwork component; yet in reality, code blue situations involve all members of the health care team. Their program engages interprofessional teams to participate in the training together and uses equipment that is onsite, accessible, and utilized by actual teams in their clinical setting. These two fellowship participants recognized that staff comfort levels, ability to use emergency supplies, and ability to work efficiently as a team all have the potential to increase patient safety and increase positive resuscitation outcomes. Their fellowship is complete and their program has gained organizational recognition and support and is now being implemented in other areas.

Another example of a successful project is a pain management initiative led by a registered practical nurse (equivalent to an LPN or LVN outside of Ontario) who developed and implemented an evidence-informed interprofessional education program focused on assessment, pain management strategies, documentation, interprofessional collaboration, and patient education to improve pain management for patients in rehabilitation. This nurse noticed that patients were not always able to complete all of their daily rehabilitation activities because of pain. Through this fellowship opportunity she was able to investigate this further; she found that each profession working with these patients was approaching pain management through their own professional lens. Once she brought the team together, they were able to find collaborative approaches to improve pain management for their patients. This work has helped support patients to be able to fully participate in and complete their rehabilitation activities and improve their quality of life.

Multiple factors have contributed to the success of the CAP Fellowship Program. Each participant receives mentoring, coaching, and support from their managers, mentors, and program faculty. The weekly fellowship seminars, which are facilitated by the faculty, also provide an opportunity and safe space for participants to share their successes and challenges and to engage in dialogue with one another and the faculty to help identify ways to overcome challenges and navigate systems, organizational politics, and other complexities. Part of this includes learning how to present their ideas to leaders and other stakeholders in a way that captures their attention and interest, as well as how to engage their colleagues in a way that facilitates a sense of ownership among them.

It also includes coaching to help them explore and consider multiple perspectives, particularly in situations in which they may encounter what might be perceived as resistance or pushback from others in the organization. This coaching helps them look beyond the surface to understand the reasons for this resistance, and they are then able to address those issues constructively for a positive outcome. Interprofessional collaboration also plays a big role in their success; each year, participants from a variety of professions learn with, from, and about one another as they lead their improvement projects. This helps participants to see things from a variety of perspectives they may not have considered before, and it helps them expand their network to include multiple professions across the organization. It also helps them to lead for interprofessional collaboration—and essentially good teamwork—with their point-of-care colleagues on a day-to-day basis.

The CAP Fellowship Program also depends on a particular style of leadership for its success. The most meaningful and critical change needs to come from and be led by those who are engaged directly with our patients; this can only occur if there is support from formal organizational leaders at the top level. UHN's leaders have fostered an environment that enables this type of grassroots approach to improving patient care. They have also found ways to identify financial resources to support the protected time for the participants in the CAP Fellowship Program; although this is an ongoing challenge each year, the growing success of the program is helping demonstrate its value to potential funders. Support has come from a variety of sources, including our nursing and health professions leaders, clinical program leaders, physician leaders, and our Foundation.

Excellence in patient care is everybody's business, and it relies on ongoing evaluation of and improvements to the way we do things. Hospitals all over the world are struggling to find ways to improve the patient experience by reducing medical errors and injuries, eliminating inefficiencies, and increasing employee engagement. One way to do this is to tap into the knowledge, expertise, and leadership abilities of health professionals at the point of care and to leverage good teamwork to facilitate positive change. Bringing quality improvement and change to life and sustaining the forward momentum is a complex, multifaceted endeavor that relies on the ongoing courage, commitment, and contributions of all our point-of-care teams and those who support them. The CAP Fellowship Program has created a profound shift for health professionals at the point of care and has proven to be a powerful model for achieving revolutionary change to the way we approach care. It marks a new era of meaningful, sustainable improvement in health care.

· · ·

CAROLYN PLUMMER, RN, MHSc is Senior Manager of Innovation for Collaborative Academic Practice at University Health Network in Toronto and Adjunct Lecturer at the Lawrence S. Bloomberg Faculty of Nursing at the University of Toronto. Her work focuses on leadership, innovative care models, quality improvement, and healthy work environments. She established a fellowship program aimed at supporting health care professionals to lead innovative quality improvement projects at the point of care; this program has been awarded a leading practice designation by Accreditation Canada. She is currently completing a doctoral program at Fielding Graduate University.

JOY RICHARDS, RN, PhD is the Vice-President Health Professions and Chief Nursing Executive at University Health Network (UHN) in Toronto.

She is a past president of the Academy of Canadian Executive Nurses (ACEN) and holds clinical appointments at the Lawrence S. Bloomberg Faculty of Nursing at the University of Toronto, York University Faculty of Nursing, and Humber College. She leads patient-centered care, provides strategic direction for practice, education and research, and promotes shared leadership for health professions at UHN.

"Co" Is Cool

Suzanne Gordon and Rebecca Shunk

Health care is obsessed with leadership. Go to any website of any health care professional school and you will find that that school—whether of medicine, dentistry, nursing, or any other of the professions—is training "future leaders." Schools of nursing and other professional schools have courses on leadership. Books abound that teach people to be leaders of teams, of groups, of hospitals, and of businesses. But how is leadership defined? Whether on a hospital unit or at an institution or systemwide level, leadership is too often defined as "I tell you what to do, and you do it" or "I make you think you want to do what I want you to do, and you do it." A leader is therefore a person who acts on, not with, others. Indeed, in our society, the leader is conceptualized as "the decider"—as one US president put it not so long ago. Leadership is thus a singular not a group action, an individual endeavor not a collaborative one. Of course, someone does have to make sure decisions are made and implemented, but on a team, the question is not only who makes those decisions but also how they are made. This, of course, affects whether anyone will follow the leader, which, in turn, determines whether the person who is declared to be a leader is in fact doing any leading. As Robert Ginnett has pointed out, you cannot be a leader if no one is following you. You may be a prophet, ahead of the curve, a visionary, a pioneer, or perhaps even a positive deviant but if you are alone on the battlefield, the office, the hospital or clinic, a leader is something you most definitely are not.[11]

Leading *with* other people is not something that is usually taught in our culture. Leadership as job sharing (not as job extending, as in physician-extender or job delegating) is simply not a usual part of the job description of being a leader in health care or anywhere else. If we do not begin to define leadership as something one sometimes does *with* someone else, rather than *to* someone else, how can we engage in collaborative or interprofessional work?

We began to reflect on this question in conversations we had together in fall 2013 when we were asked to lead a faculty-development session in interprofessional education at the University of California, San Francisco. We'd never met before and had only a few weeks to plan our class, prepare the PowerPoint, and then lead the two-hour session.

As a physician at the VA (Rebecca) and a journalist/health care observer for almost thirty years (Suzanne), we discovered we had a lot to talk about when it came to developing our presentation on teamwork and creating some sort of team-based intervention for an interprofessional education (IPE) program. As we talked about good and poor teamwork and communication and the challenges faced in health care, we quickly moved from the intellectual to the personal. Rebecca confessed that one of her professional and personal challenges was to move from the academic model of individual achievement and advancement to a more collective, collaborative mode. When Suzanne asked her what she meant, she told the following story.

Rebecca is a primary care provider, educator, and physician codirector of the Center of Excellence (COE) in Primary Care Education at the San Francisco VA Medical Center. She and an interprofessional team try to develop innovative strategies to improve education for interprofessional team-based health professions in patient-centered primary care. For several years Rebecca had waited to gather enough results to present the center's work at a high-stakes presentation—medical grand rounds. This venue provides a weekly opportunity for University of California, San Francisco, faculty to present their academic work for peer review.

Grand rounds are a milestone on the way toward academic advancement and peer acceptance for a professor. Rebecca remembers, "Despite the fact that I had become a leader in IPE and teamwork, I pressed on in a singular quest to tackle the data of our center and develop a PowerPoint presentation that would wow my colleagues with 'my' work. I remember the day that Terry Keene, a seasoned nurse practitioner who had been newly appointed to serve with me as codirector of the center, asked me what I was working on. Only then did it dawn on me that I had not included her in the presentation of our work. The topic was 'interprofessional collaboration' of all things! Did I really not think of asking her to copresent?

"Despite all of my teamwork and collaboration flag waving I had clearly not fully embraced the co-director role. I was barreling ahead as the 'director' with no more insight than other uninformed providers I had worked hard to educate. My actions were a real eye-opener to me. The more I thought about what got me to this place the more it became clear: 'co' is not cool. 'Co,' although key to everything we are teaching our trainees about IPE, is not the currency of our promotional process. Being the director, not the co-director, is the path to professorship. Because I had built an open relationship with Terry, I was able to admit my misstep and at the same time acknowledge the fact that in academic medicine we have yet to change the currency. This is but one more hurdle we have to tackle for true interprofessional collaboration in the academic health care setting."

As Suzanne listened to Rebecca's story, she recognized familiar themes. Although Suzanne doesn't work in an academic health care setting, she is the coeditor of an academic series on health care for Cornell University Press (including this book). Suzanne looked a bit sheepish and had to confess that she had a "co" problem as well. Suzanne coedits the series along with Sioban Nelson, who is vice provost for Academic Affairs at of the University of Toronto. When Suzanne approaches authors or the media or faculty about her books, she always presents herself as coeditor of the Culture and Politics of Health Care Work book series. There are times, however, Suzanne also confessed, when this "co" business presents a dilemma. "I have to admit," she said, "that when I'm approaching a well-known author or journalist I find myself tempted to say or write 'editor' rather than 'coeditor.' It's as though being a cosomething is less valuable than being the sole authority, decider, or main character on the stage. In our culture, when you're a co, you're not the star. You fear you will have less authority, get less respect, and be considered less valuable. Who would want to play with a co? So I have to struggle against my inclination to introduce myself as 'editor of the series' and to continually emphasize that I am coeditor, which is what I am."

We both agreed that we had to grapple with the socially constructed tendency to put ourselves up front rather than share our leadership roles. Co, we agreed, is simply not considered to be cool. As we discussed our presentation to the faculty, we decided that we had to include this dilemma. To really lead teams and be members of teams we have to change the dynamics of cool. Co has to become cool. We decided not only to talk about this in class but to try to do a slide or poster on the subject. We went home to the dictionary and looked up all the "co" words we could find. So many of the words we use in common parlance—like common—are "co" words. They reflect the fact that human beings actually live in community—another "co" word, that we do things not just to other people but with them. Here is what we came up with.

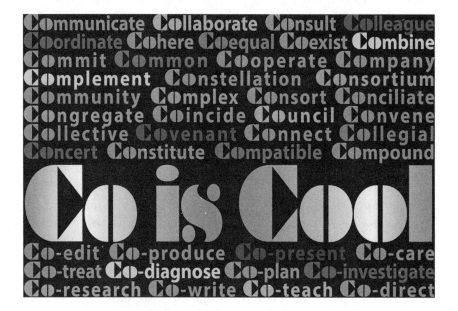

Notes

INTRODUCTION

1. Institute of Medicine, *To Err Is Human: Building a Safer Health System* (Washington, DC: National Academy Press, 1999).

2. Institute of Medicine, Committee on Quality of Health Care in America, *Crossing the Quality Chasm: A New Health System for the 21st Century* (Washington, DC: National Academy Press, 2001).

3. World Health Organization, "Framework for Action on Interprofessional Education and Collaborative Practice," http://www.who.int/hrh/re sources/framework_action/en (accessed June 19, 2013); J. Frenk, I. Chen, Z. Bhutta, J. Cohen, N. Crips, T. Evans, H. Fineberg, P. Garcia, Y. Ke, B. Kistnasamy, A. Meleis, D. Naylor, A. Pablos-Mendex, S. Reddy, S. Scrimshaw, J. Sepulveda, D. Serwadda, and H. Zurayk, "Health Professionals for a New Century: Transforming Education to Strengthen Health Systems in an Interdependent World," *Lancet* 376 (2010): 1923–58.

4. Suzanne Gordon. *Nursing against the Odds: How Health Care Cost Cutting, Media Stereotypes, and Medical Hubris Undermine Nurses and Patient Care* (Ithaca: Cornell University Press, 2005).

5. John T. James, "A New Evidence-Based Estimate of Patient Harms Associated with Hospital Care," *Journal of Patient Safety* 9, no. 3: 122–28.

6. Erving Goffman, *Presentation of Self in Everyday Life* (Garden City, NY: Doubleday Anchor, 1959).

7. J. Richard Hackman, Harvard Business School, *Working Knowledge*, "Leading Teams," http://hbswk.hbs.edu/archive/2996.html (accessed June 3, 2012).

8. J. Richard Hackman, ed., *Groups That Work (and Those That Don't): Creating Conditions for Effective Teamwork* (San Francisco, CA: Jossey-Bass, 1990), 6–7.

9. C. Guglielmi, D. L. Feldman, A. P. Marco, P. Graling, M. Hoppes, L. L. Asplin, and L. Groah, "Defining Competency in High-Performance Teams," *AORN Journal* 93, no. 5: 528–38.

10. Scott Reeves, Simon Lewin, Sherry Espin, and Merrick Zwarenstein, *Interprofessional Teamwork for Health and Social Care* (Oxford, UK: John Wiley & Sons, 2010).

11. Suzanne Gordon, "On Teams, Teamwork, and Team Intelligence," in *First, Do Less Harm: Confronting the Inconvenient Problems of Patient Safety*, ed. Ross Koppel and Suzanne Gordon (Ithaca: Cornell University Press, 2012), 196–220.

12. Edgar H. Schein, *Helping: How to Offer, Give, and Receive Help* (San Francisco, CA: Berrett-Koehler, 2011), 3.

13. Edwin Hutchins, *Cognition in the Wild* (Cambridge: MIT Press, 1995).

14. *Strategy + Business*, Interview with Chris Argyris, http://www.strategy-business.com/article/9887?gko=c19c5 (accessed June 15, 2013).

15. Edgar H. Schein and Warren G. Bennis, *Personal and Organizational Change through Group Methods* (New York: Wiley, 1965), 44–45.

16. Amy C. Edmondson, "Managing the Risk of Learning: Psychological Safety in Work Teams," in *International Handbook of Organizational Teamwork and Cooperative Learning*, ed. M. A. West, D. Tjosvold, and K. G. Smith (New York: Wiley, 2003), 258.

17. Robert Ginnett, "Crews as Groups: Their Formation and Their Leadership," in *Cockpit Resource Management*, ed. Earl L. Weiner, Barbara G. Kanki, and Robert L. Helmreich (Amsterdam: Academic Press, 1993), 84.

PART 1

1. David P. Baker, Sigrid Gustafson, Jeff Beaubien, Eduardo Salas, and Paul Barach, *Medical Teamwork and Patient Safety: The Evidence-Based Relation*, report prepared for the James Battles Center for Quality Improvement and Patient Safety, Agency for Healthcare Research and Quality (AHRQ), Rockville, Maryland, October 20, 2003.

2. Institute of Medicine, *To Err Is Human: Building a Safer Health System* (Washington, DC: National Academies Press, 1999).

3. D. C. Classen, R. Resar, F. Griffin, F. Federico, T. Frankel, N. Kimmel, J. C. Whittington, A. Frankel A, Seger, and B. C. James, "'Global Trigger Tool' Shows That Adverse Events in Hospitals May Be Ten Times Greater Than Previously Measured," *Health Affairs* 30 (April 2011): 4, 1–9.

4. For an excellent discussion of the concept of "mature leadership," see Robert C. Ginnett, "Crews as Groups: Their Formation and Their Leadership,"

in *Cockpit Resource Management*, ed. Earl L. Wiener, Barbara G. Kanki, and Robert L. Helmreich (San Diego, CA: Academic Press, 1993), 84. Also see Joseph P. Dunlop and Susan J. Mangold, *Leadership/Followership Recurrent Training Instructor Manual* (Washington, DC: Office of the Chief Scientific and Technical Advisor for Human Factors to the Federal Aviation Administration [AAR-100], 1998), 44, www.crm-devel.org/ftp/instman.pdf (accessed April 12, 2013).

5. Agency for Health Care Research and Quality, Department of Defense, *TeamSTEPPS Instructor Guide*, Evidence Base: Mutual Support.

6. "SBAR Technique for Communication: A Situation Briefing Model," Institute for Health Care Improvement, http://www.ihi.org/knowledge/Pages/Tools/SBARTechniqueforCommunicationASituationalBriefingModel.aspx (accessed July 8, 2011). In this book, see part 4 "Getting Help When You Need It" and part 8 "The Devil's in the Details" for a discussion of SBAR.

7. A. Tucker and A. Edmondson, "Why Hospitals Don't Learn from Failures: Organizational and Psychological Dynamics That Inhibit System Change," working paper, Harvard Business School, November 6, 2002.

8. Karl E. Weick, Kathleen M. Suttcliffe, and David Obstfeld, "Organizing for High Reliability: Processes of Collective Mindfulness," in *Research in Organizational Behavior*, vol. 1, ed. R. S. Sutton and B. M. Shaw (Stanford: Jal Press, 1999),81–123. accessed December 12, 2013, http://www.drillscience.com/DPS/Organizing%20for%20High%20Reliability.pdf.

9. Chesley Sullenberger, personal communication to Suzanne Gordon, August 13, 2013.

PART 2

1. J. A. Janocha and R. T. Smith, *Workplace Safety and Health in the Health Care and Social Assistance Industry* (Washington, DC: Bureau of Labor Statistics, 2010), www.bls.gov/opub/cwc/sh20100825ar01p1.htm (accessed April 8, 2013); Linda A. Treiber and Jackie H. Jones, "Wounds That Don't Heal: Nurses' Experience with Medication Errors," in *First, Do Less Harm: Confronting the Inconvenient Problems of Patient Safety*, ed. Ross Koppel and Suzanne Gordon (Ithaca: Cornell University Press, 2012), 150–79.

2. Robert. M. Sapolsky, *Why Zebras Don't Get Ulcers* (New York: Holt, 2004).

3. "The Silent Treatment: Why Safety Tools and Checklists Aren't Enough to Save Lives," VitalSmarts 2011, http://www.silencetreatmentstudy.com (accessed January 20, 2014).

4. Suzanne Gordon, Patrick Mendenhall, and Bonnie O'Connor, *Beyond the Checklist: What Else Health Care Can Learn from Aviation Teamwork and Safety* (Ithaca: Cornell University Press, 2012), 16–17.

5. Diane Vaughan, *The Challenger Launch Decision: Risk, Technology, Culture, and Deviance at NASA* (Chicago: University of Chicago Press, 1996), xiv.

6. Paul Rozin and Edward B. Royzman, "Negativity Bias, Negativity Dominance, and Contagion," *Personality and Social Psychology Review* 5, no. 4 (2001): 296–320.

7. Mark Singer, "Task Saturation, Ruthless Ignorance, and the Power of Focus," *No Map. No Guide. No Limits* (blog), March 23, 2010, http://www.nomap noguidenolimits.com/2010/03/23/task-saturation/ (accessed April 14, 2014).

8. The Leapfrog Group, "Half of US Hospitals Reporting to Leapfrog Say They Won't Bill for a Never Event, press release, September 26, 2007, http://www.leapfroggroup.org/media/file/Release_-_Adoption_of_Leapfrog_Never_Events_Policy_2007.pdf (accessed June 15, 2013).

PART 3

1. Susan Edgman Levitan, "Involving the Patient in Safety Efforts," in *Achieving Safe and Reliable Health Care: Strategies and Solutions*, ed. Michael S. Leonard, Allan Frankel, Terri Simmonds, and Kathleen B. Vega (Chicago: Health Administration Press, 2004), 81–92.

2. Leonard L. Berry and Neeli Bendapudi, "Clueing In Customers," *Harvard Business Review* 81, no. 2 (February 2003): 100–106, 126.

3. Dominick L. Frosch, Suepattra G. May, Katharine A. S. Rendle, Caroline Tietbohl, and Glyn Elwynet, "Authoritarian Physicians and Patients Fear of Being Labeled 'Difficult' among Key Obstacles to Shared Decision Making," *Health Affairs* 31, no. 5 (2012): 1030–38; PIPS (Patient Involvement in Patient Safety) Group, "Speaking Up about Safety Concerns and Experiences: Multi-Setting Qualitative Study of Patients' Views." *Quality and Safety in Health Care* 19, no. 6 (2010): 1–7.

4. Donald M. Berwick, *Escape Fire: Designs for the Future of Health Care* (San Francisco, CA: Jossey-Bass, 2003).

5. Edward E. Rosenbaum, *A Taste of My Own Medicine: When the Doctor Is the Patient* (New York: Random House, 1988); Jody Heymann, *Equal Partners: A Physician's Call for a New Spirit of Medicine* (Philadelphia: University of Pennsylvania Press, 2000).

6. Arnold Relman, "On Breaking One's Neck," *New York Review of Books*, February 6, 2014, http://www.nybooks.com/articles/archives/2014/feb/06/on-breaking-ones-neck/ (accessed February 20, 2014).

7. The Diabetes Control and Complications Trial Research Group, "The Effect of Intensive Treatment of Diabetes on the Development and Progression of Long-Term Complications in Insulin-Dependent Diabetes Mellitus," *New England Journal of Medicine* 329 (1993): 977–86.

8. Ibid.

9. A. Bandura. "Self-efficacy: Toward a Unifying Theory of Behavioral Change," *Psychological Review* 84 (1977): 191–215.

10. E. H. Wagner, et al. "Improving Chronic Illness Care: Translating Evidence into Action," *Health Affairs* (Millwood) 20 (2001): 64–78.

11. D. L. Frosch, S. G. May, K. A. S. Rendle, C. Tietbohl, and G. Elwyn, "Authoritarian Physicians and Patients' Fear of Being Labeled 'Difficult' among Key Obstacles to Shared Decision Making," *Health Affairs* (Millwood) 31 (2012): 1030–38.

12. The Diabetes Control and Complications Trial Research Group, "The Effect of Intensive Treatment of Diabetes on the Development and Progression of Long-Term Complications in Insulin-Dependent Diabetes Mellitus," *New England Journal of Medicine* 329 (1993): 977–86.

13. D. L. Frosch, S. G. May, K. A. S. Rendle, C. Tietbohl, and G. Elwyn, "Authoritarian Physicians and Patients' Fear of Being Labeled 'Difficult' among Key Obstacles to Shared Decision Making," *Health Affairs* (Millwood) 31 (2012): 1030–38.

PART 4

1. Agnes Bognár, Paul Barach, Julie K. Johnson, Robert C. Duncan, David Birnbach, Donna Woods, Jane L. Holl, and Emile A. Bacha, "Errors and the Burden of Errors: Attitudes, Perceptions, and the Culture of Safety in Pediatric Cardiac Surgical Teams," *Annals of Thoracic Surgery* 85, no. 4 (April 2008): 1374–81.

2. AHRQ, "Chart 5–4. Average Percentage of Respondents Reporting Events in the Past 12 Months, across All 2012 Database Hospitals: Hospital Survey on Patient Safety Culture: 2012 User Comparative Database Report," December 2012, Agency for Healthcare Research and Quality, Rockville, MD, http://www.ahrq.gov/professionals/quality-patient-safety/patientsafetyculture/hospital/2012/hosp12chart5-4.html (accessed November 17, 2013).

3. J. B. Sexton, M. A. Makary, A. R. Tersigni, D. Pryor, A. Hendrich, E. J. Thomas, C. G. Holzmueller, A. P. Knight, Y. Wu, and P. J. Pronovost, "Teamwork in the Operating Room: Frontline Perspectives among Hospitals and Operating Room Personnel," *Anesthesiology* 105, no. 5 (November 2006): 877–84.

4. Linda Flynn, "The State of the Nursing Workforce in New Jersey: Findings from a Statewide Survey of Registered Nurses" (Newark: New Jersey Collaborating Center for Nursing, 2007), 19.

5. Lucian L. Leape, Miles F. Shore, Jules L. Dienstag, Robert J. Mayer, Susan Edgman-Levitan, Gregg S. Meyer, and Gerald B. Healy, "Perspective: A Culture of Respect, Part 1: The Nature and Causes of Disrespect by Physicians," *Academic Medicine* 87, no. 7 (July 2012): 1, accessed June 2, 2012, http://journals.lww.com/academicmedicine/Abstract/publishahead/Perspective.

6. Lucian Leape Institute, *Through the Eyes of the Workforce: Creating Joy, Meaning, and Safer Health Care*, report of the Roundtable on Joy and Meaning in Work and Workforce Safety (Boston: National Patient Safety Foundation, 2013), 5.

7. J. Bryan Sexton, Eric J. Thomas, and Robert L. Helmreich, "Error, Stress, and Teamwork in Medicine and Aviation: Cross Sectional Surveys," *Journal of Human Performance in Extreme Environments* 6, no. 1 (December 2001).

8. Anita L. Tucker and Amy C. Edmondson, "Why Hospitals Don't Learn from Failures: Organizational and Psychological Dynamics That Inhibit System Change," *California Management Review* 45, no 2 (2003): 63.

9. Ibid.

PART 5

1. J. Richard Hackman and Ruth Wageman, "A Theory of Team Coaching," *Academy of Management Review* 30, no 2 (2005): 269–87, accessed December 27, 2013, http://nolostcapital.com/sites/nolostcapital.nl/files/blog-attachments/Publicatie_A_Theory_of_Team_Coaching.pdf.

2. Ibid., 283.

3. Chris Chen, *Coaching Training* (Alexandria, VA: ASTD Press, 2003).

4. Anita L. Tucker and Amy C. Edmondson, "Why Hospitals Don't Learn from Failures: Organizational and Psychological Dynamics That Inhibit System Change," *California Management Review* 45, no. 2 (2003): 63.

5. Amy C. Edmondson, "Managing the Risk of Learning: Psychological Safety in Work Teams," in *International Handbook of Organizational Teamwork and Cooperative Learning*, ed. M. A. West, D. Tjosvold, and K. G. Smith (New York: Wiley, 2003), 258.

6. Anita L. Tucker and Amy C. Edmondson, "Why Hospitals Don't Learn from Failures: Organizational and Psychological Dynamics That Inhibit System Change," *California Management Review* 45, no. 2 (2003): 60.

PART 6

1. *Silence Kills: The Seven Crucial Conversations for Healthcare* (American Association of Critical Care Nurses and Vital Smarts Industry Watch, 2005),

http://www.aacn.org/WD/practice/docs/publicpolicy/silencekills.pdf (accessed June 9, 2011).

2. Suzanne Gordon, Patrick Mendenhall, and Bonnie Blair O'Connor, *Beyond the Checklist: What Else Health Care Can Learn from Aviation Teamwork and Safety* (Ithaca: Cornell University Press, 2012), 185.

PART 7

1. World Health Organization, Health Professions Networks Nursing and Midwifery Office, Department of Human Resources for Health, "Framework for Action on Interprofessional Education and Collaborative Practice," Geneva, Switzerland, 2010, http://whqlibdoc.who.int/hq/2010/WHO_HRH_HPN_10.3_eng.pdf, (accessed January 2, 2014).

2. Thomas J. Nasca, Ingrid Philibert, Timothy Brigham, and Timothy C. Flynn, "The Next GME Accreditation System—Rationale and Benefits," *New England Journal of Medicine* 366 (March 15, 2012): 1051–56.

3. American College of Graduate Medical Education, "Interprofessional Core Competencies," *GME Today* 6, no 12 (December 2011), http://www.gmetoday.org/gmeconnections/937/Interprofessional_Core_Competencies (accessed January 2, 2014).

4. The Interprofessional Education Collaborative (IPEC) website can be found at https://ipecollaborative.org.

5. Alison M. Trinkoff and Jeanne Geiger-Brown, "Sleep Deprived Nurses: Sleep and Schedule Challenges in Nursing," in *First, Do Less Harm: Confronting the Inconvenient Problems of Patient Safety*, ed. Ross Koppel and Suzanne Gordon (Ithaca: Cornell University Press, 2012), 168–79.

6. Barbara J. Safriet, "Health Care Dollars and Regulatory Sense: The Role of Advanced Practice Nursing," Faculty Scholarship Series Paper 4423, *Yale Journal on Regulation* 9 (1992): 417–88.

7. Institute of Medicine, *Crossing the Quality Chasm: A New Health System for the 21st Century* (Washington, DC: National Academy Press, 2001), 68.

PART 8

1. Delos M. Cosgrove, Michael Fisher, Patricia Gabow, Gary Gottlieb, George C. Halvorson, Brent C. James, Gary S. Kaplan, Jonathan B. Perlin, Robert Petzel, Glenn D. Steele, and John S. Toussaint, "Ten Strategies to Lower Costs, Improve Quality, and Engage Patients: The View from Leading Health System CEOs," *Health Affairs* 32, no. 2 (2013): 321–27.

2. Richard Pascale, Jerry Sternin, and Monique Sternin, *The Power of Positive Deviance: How Unlikely Innovators Solve the World's Toughest Problems* (Cambridge: Harvard Business Review Press, 2010).

3. Karl E. Weick and Kathleen M. Sutcliffe, *Managing the Unexpected: Resilient Performance in an Age of Uncertainty* (San Francisco, CA: Jossey-Bass, 2008).

4. See also, Rajiv Jain, Stephen M. Kralovic, Martin E. Evans, Meredith Ambrose, Loretta A. Simbartl, Scott Obrosky, Marta L. Render, Ron W. Freyberg, John A. Jernigan, Robert R. Muder, LaToya J. Miller, and Gary A. Roselle, "Veterans Affairs Initiative to Prevent Methicillan-Resistant *Staphylococcus aureus* Infections," *New England Journal of Medicine* 364 (April 14, 2011): 1419–30.

5. Peter Lazes, Suzanne Gordon, and Sameh Samy, "Excluded Actors in Patient Safety," in *First, Do Less Harm: Confronting the Inconvenient Problems of Patient Safety*, ed. Ross Koppel and Suzanne Gordon (Ithaca, N.Y.: Cornell University Press, 2012), 93–122.

6. University of Texas, Center for Healthcare Quality and Safety, Safety Attitudes and Safety Climate Questionnaire, https://med.uth.edu/chqs/surveys/safety-attitudes-and-safety-climate-questionnaire/ (accessed July 20, 2013).

7. Michael Block et al., "The Tangible Handoff: A Team Approach for Advancing Structured Communication in Labor and Delivery," *The Joint Commission Journal on Quality and Patient Safety* 36, no. 6 (June 2010): 282–87.

8. NPSF white paper.

9. Alex B. Haynes, Thomas G. Weiser, William R. Berry, Stuart R. Lipsitz, Abdel-Hadi S. Breizat, E. Patchen Dellinger, Teodoro Herbosa, Sudhir Joseph, Pascience L. Kibatala, Marie Carmela M. Lapitan, Alan F. Merry, Krishna Moorthy, Richard K. Reznick, Bryce Taylor, and Atul A. Gawande, "Safe Surgery Saves Lives Study Group: A Surgical Safety Checklist to Reduce Morbidity and Mortality in a Global Population," *New England Journal of Medicine* 360, no. 5 (2009): 491–99.

10. Julia Neily, Peter D. Mills, Yinong Young-Xu, Brian T. Carney, Priscilla West, David H. Berger, Lisa M. Mazzia, Douglas E. Paull, and James P. Bagian, "Association between Implementation of a Medical Team Training Program and Surgical Mortality," *JAMA* 304, no. 15 (2010): 1693–1700.

11. Robert C. Ginnett, "Crews as Groups: Their Formation and Their Leadership," in *Cockpit Resource Management*, ed. Earl L. Wiener, Barbara G. Kanki, and Robert L. Helmreich (San Diego: Academic Press, 1993), 84.

Editors

SUZANNE GORDON is an award-winning journalist and author who writes about health care delivery, health care systems, and patient safety. Her eighteen books include *First, Do Less Harm: Confronting the Inconvenient Problems of Patient Safety*. Her latest book is *Beyond the Checklist: What Else Health Care Can Learn from Aviation Teamwork and Safety*. Her books on health care have been published by Cornell University Press in the Culture and Politics of Health Care Work series, which she coedits. She has been a commentator for CBS radio and National Public Radio's *Marketplace*. Her articles have appeared in *Harper's*, the *Atlantic*, the *New York Times* and the *New York Times Magazine*, the *Los Angeles Times*, the *Boston Globe*, the *Toronto Globe and Mail*, and many other publications. She is also coauthor, with Lisa Hayes, of *Bedside Manners*, a play about team relationships in health care that has been performed at numerous venues including the Institute for Healthcare Improvement, the Hospital of the University of Pennsylvania, and Cedars-Sinai Medical Center. It is being used in interprofessional education programs in the United States and Canada, including the University of Toronto and the University of California, San Francisco (UCSF). The play and accompanying workbook are published by Cornell University Press. She is a Visiting Professor at the University of Maryland School of Nursing and Assistant Adjunct Professor at the UCSF School of Nursing. She is also an Affiliated Scholar at the Wilson Centre at the University of Toronto's Faculty of Medicine and a Visiting Scholar at the Center for Innovation in Interprofessional Education at UCSF. She is an editorial board member of the *Journal of Interprofessional Care*.

DAVID L. FELDMAN, MD is Senior Vice President and Chief Medical Officer at Hospitals Insurance Company, which provides professional liability for hospitals, physicians, and health care professionals throughout New

York State. He is responsible for risk management activities and works on innovative programs aimed at improving patient safety and quality of care. Previously, he was Vice President for Patient Safety, Vice President of Perioperative Services, and Vice Chairman of the Department of Surgery at Maimonides Medical Center in Brooklyn. He implemented numerous patient safety initiatives including the use of the WHO surgical checklist. Formerly President of the Maimonides Medical Staff, he was instrumental in the creation and implementation of the hospital-wide Code of Mutual Respect and the physician peer review committee. He has served on the American College of Surgeons (ACS) Committee on Perioperative Care and as Vice Chairman of the ACS Collaborative Task Force for the development of high-performance teams in surgery. He also served as the ACS liaison to the AORN Recommended Practices Committee. He is a master Team-STEPPS trainer and a certified trainer in Crucial Conversations and Crucial Confrontations. He received a bachelor's degree and MD from Duke University and completed Plastic Surgery training at Duke University Medical Center. He earned an MBA from the NYU Stern School of Business and is a Certified Physician Executive.

MICHAEL LEONARD, MD is Managing Partner of Safe and Reliable Healthcare, Adjunct Professor of Medicine at Duke University, and a faculty member at the Institute for Healthcare Improvement. He has helped train over 1,500 patient safety officers through the IHI Executive Patient Safety Officer Course. He was formerly the National Physician Leader for Patient Safety at Kaiser Permanente. A Cardiac Anesthesiologist by training, he has been active in applying high-reliability principles for other high-risk industries into health care. For the past decade, he has taught extensively throughout the Kaiser system and outside organizations within North America and the United Kingdom, with a focus on surgical safety, obstetrics, and critical care. He has a particular interest in safety culture and the organizational factors that enhance effective teamwork and safer care in complex environments.